Hormone Heresy

WHAT WOMEN <u>MUST</u> KNOW ABOUT THEIR HORMONES

by Sherrill Sellman

D0054941

GetWell International

GetWell International, Inc
350 Ward Avenue - Suite 106
Honolulu, Hawaii   USA - 96814
eMail: golight@aloha.net

(ISBN 0-958-72520-9)

Production & Cover graphics by: GetWell Designs

Photo Credit: Dennis Ryan - Melbourne Australia

USA Distribution: BookWorld Companies - 1933 Whitfield Park Loop
                    Sarasota, FL 34243

Order Fulfillment: 1 800 444-2524 ext 225

Printed by: Quebecor Printing Book Group,
                    New York, New York, 10022-6824 USA

Linda,

Always
honor the
wisdom of
your feminine Self.

Shemiel

Contents

Part One –
The Untold Hormone Story

Chapter   1

Chapter   2

Chapter   3

Chapter   4

Chapter   5

Chapter 5 (cont)

Chapter 6

Chapter 7

Chapter 8

Chapter 9

Chapter 10

Chapter 11

Chapter 12

Chapter 13

Chapter 14

Chapter 15

Chapter 15 (cont)

Chapter 16

Chapter 17

Chapter 18

Chapter 19

Chapter 20

Part Two —
The Journey to Hell and Back

Part Three —
The Feminine Path to Power

Chapter 1

Chapter 2

Chapter 3

Part Four —
Returning to Balance

Chapter 1

Chapter 2

Chapter 3

Chapter 4

Chapter 5

Chapter 6

Chapter 7

Chapter 8

Chapter 9

Chapter 10

Chapter 11

Foreword:

Like most women, Sherrill Sellman sailed through her first four decades of life with little knowledge and certainly no concern about the hormones which feminize our bodies. However, as women on the eve of the third millennium have discovered, modern mid-life brings new perceptions of hormones. Women with menopausal bodies are now the hot property of an industry which is dominated by medically prescribed hormones. Prominently displayed on pharmacy shelves, menopause hormones are touted as the answer to the physical and emotional signals of a woman's fading youth - creased and thinning skin, bone loss, declining sexual appetite and so on. Heart attacks, strokes, hip fractures and senility are supposedly the stuff of women from a past and unenlightened age. In other words, medicine has conquered aging and provides women with the key to an eternal prime. Extrapolating from the menopause fraternity's ever-expanding cure all claims of hormone replacement therapy [HRT], cancer appears to be the last remaining barrier between women and immortality.

Yet, as Professor of Community Medicine at Sydney's Manly Hospital, Deborah Saltman describes in her 1994 volume, *In Transition, A Guide to Menopause*, the HRT fix can leave menopausal women prisoners of their own and their doctor's making. Put another way, the HRT cure can be worse than the ailment. Equally, it is crucial to remember that the overwhelming majority of menopausal women opting to travel down the HRT pathway are doing so in the absence of signs or symptoms of age-related disorders. Only a minority of women commence HRT to relieve their mid-life discomfort from hot flushes, vaginal dryness and lethargy. Rather, the overall majority opt for HRT on the basis of a medically promised future which is devoid of heart disease, stroke, osteoporosis and

Alzheimer's disease. In general, the dogma of the menopausal hormone brigade was developed by a male fraternity of medical professionals. Over the past decade, eminent authors from Germaine Greer to Betty Friedan and Sandra Coney have voiced their criticism and concern about the hormonal hype which has dominated perceptions of what amounts to good medicine for menopausal women. Even as the debates still rage over whether HRT increases the risk of breast cancer and worsens existing complaints such as migraine, varicose veins and the like, dissenting medical opinion is less visible. Nonetheless, it does exist. Epidemiologist Elizabeth Barrett-Connor has argued for more than a decade that there is but thin evidence to support the prevailing medical philosophy that HRT prevents women's heart disease. Bone biologists, too, are wary of both HRT and calcium cures for osteoporosis stressing that: .....the effects of estrogen deficiency have been overemphasized, ... factors relating to socio-economic development may be more important than estrogen deficiency to the pathogenesis of osteoporosis, and calcium is a nutrient, not a drug. The only disorder it can be expected to alleviate is calcium deficiency.

The World Health Organization has emphasized the need for research to explain the increased incidence of unexpected death of venous thromboembolism in women prescribed synthetic progestin contraceptives. However, progestins commonly in the form of medroxyprogesterone bearing the trade name of Provera, are frequently prescribed in HRT protocols to counteract the increased risk of endometrial cancer from estrogen when taken alone. Vindicating past warnings, alarming evidence surfaced in 1997 from animal studies demonstrating that medroxyprogesterone co-administered with estrogen counteracted any beneficial effects estrogen may have in preventing heart disease and stroke, and actually increased the risk of coronary vasospasm. Stressing the clinical importance of these findings, menopause experts from Wake Forest University in North Carolina warned that:

"Perfect hormone replacement therapy might be one that affords cardiovascular and bone protection without unwanted side-effects or increasing the risk of breast or uterine cancer".

Other 1997 reports confirmed the uncertainty surrounding osteoporosis-related problems with several studies suggesting that antibiotics such as Minocycline, a derivative of tetracycline, might be just as effective as HRT's estrogen in preventing the bone loss associated with osteoporosis. According to the authors of one animal study, the antibiotic probably interfered with the collagenase enzyme which is active in destroying the bone during the process of osteoporosis. Given the current problems associated with antibiotic-resistant bacteria, antibiotics are an unattractive alternative to HRT but an editorial which accompanied this research interestingly commented, "...it is hard to imagine many companies investing the millions necessary to promote it [Minocycline] to doctors and the public". Minocycline seems destined for a subordinate place in the market unless some pharmaceutical firm patents a new derivative of the drug.

In many ways, this comment and the flourish of new information casting further doubts on the HRT gospel, again raises the question of whether HRT is fueled by medical economics? In the long term, the answer is somewhat irrelevant compared with the resolution of whether HRT is, as the pro-HRT fraternity would have it, good for women? In Britain, concerned that steroidal hormones are being prescribed to women without respect for their serious side effects, a number of general medical practitioners, obstetricians and gynecologists, physicians, psychiatrists, surgeons, oncologists, radiologists, pathologists and medical scientists have formed a group known as DASH [Doctors against Abuse from Steroid sex Hormones] to educate not women but doctors about the scientific evidence of the dangers of sex hormones.

Sherrill Sellman's *Hormone Heresy* convincingly highlights the HRT bias which prevails in medical circles. As an example, it would be impossible for any self-respecting woman to altogether ignore the face value of the medical fraternity's promise that HRT decreases women's risk of heart disease. After all, women's greater life expectancy together with their steep increase in cardiac illness after menopause means that heart disease is the leading cause of death in women, accounting for one of every two female deaths and outnumbering women's total deaths from all forms of cancer. However, as recently as 1993, British clinical gerontologist Kay-Tee Khaw asked the obvious question, "where are all the women in the studies of coronary heart disease?" Khaw explained that studies wherein white middle-aged men were included, risked providing inappropriate answers for women. Sherrill too discovered that HRT is not yet imposed on white, middle-class, middle-aged men to reduce their chance of a future heart attack. Rather it is women who make up the entire HRT market, although while white, middle-class women dominated the earlier profiles of HRT users, women's well founded fear of coronary illness has enabled the menopause industry to snare less privileged, non-Caucasian women into its commercial net.

Dr. Elizabeth Barrett-Connor argues that no randomized placebo-controlled clinical trials have ever been conducted to prove that the lower incidence of heart disease in socio-economically, educationally advantaged, health conscious women is directly due to HRT. Plausibly, the diminished coronary morbidity and mortality in this group of women might equally, or otherwise, be due to their middle class privilege and their intensified medical monitoring including regular blood pressure and cholesterol measurements and general health advice, that comes with the HRT prescription. Importantly, as Barrett-Connor emphasizes, the premature appointment of HRT as women's salvation from heart disease has instead served to delay research into environmental, nutritional and life-style measures that could benefit women's hearts, bones and minds during the second half of their lives.

Sherrill Sellman's *Hormone Heresy* is an escape from the HRT penitentiary. Her approach arms women with knowledge; a precise explanation of how our hormones act in concert at different stages of our lives; the specific differences between our own human hormones and those obtained from plants, animals and the laboratories of pharmaceutical companies; an insight into the health problems ranging from the minor and transient to the severe and terminal which can arise when the fine balance between our body's natural hormone levels are disrupted by the likes of HRT.

Hormone Heresy also provides an information base about hormone-rich natural resources that can non-invasively supplement or tide us through the erratic hormonal phases that sometimes accompany the transformations of menopause. In a strong but easily understood dialogue, *Hormone Heresy* sets menopause in terms of self-help for mid-life women.

Drawing on her own research and that of others, Sherrill explains how women's personal wisdom provides a means to live an HRT-free menopause. Crucially, she reinforces the concept that menopause per se is neither a disease nor a state of decay.

In many ways, *Hormone Heresy* takes me back to Grace Paley's preface to *Women of the 14th Moon*, an anthology of North American women's stories of their menopausal experiences. Grace was referring to the laughter that met the excesses of menopausal symptoms because of the energy, risk, hope, politics, friendship and love which filled women's lives with meaning during this phase of their lives. *Hormone Heresy* fits neatly into this framework. It challenges the medical paradigm which views menopause as a process of female decomposition. *Hormone Heresy* sets the record straight - menopause is the second chapter of women's growth, one which sustains us throughout the second half of our lives.

Lynette Dumble, Ph.D. M.Sc.

Senior Research Fellow,

History and Philosophy of Science

Acknowledgements

My gratitude to my parents,
Ruth and Harry,
who nurtured my tender spirit
with love.

My gratitude to my darling husband,
James,
who always believed in me,
even when I didn't.

My gratitude to the women
throughout the world
who are following
their inner wisdom,
reclaiming their power,
speaking their truth and
giving birth to a new world.

Introduction

As I fulfil my vision of writing this book, I am driven by my passion to share with women of all ages a greater understanding of their hormonal nature and the safe alternatives that are presently available. I often posed the question to myself, "Who am I to write this book?" I am not a doctor nor a medical researcher nor do I have a string of letters after my name. Yet, as one woman in search of her truth, I realized that truth does not exclusively lie in the domain of the intellectuals or the professionals (often they are the ones most blinded by vested interests) nor in hallowed academic classrooms nor scientific laboratories. Like so many other women who are now awakening to their wise woman within, I am being guided by my intuitive wisdom not only to fulfil a greater purpose but also to speak my truth. As guardians of the sacred gift of Life, it is time for all women to courageously share their wisdom and speak up for what they believe.

My search began when it suddenly dawned upon me one day that I was rapidly approaching my menopausal years. I really hadn't thought very much about menopause—it seemed like I had years to go before I would have to deal with that mysterious 'change of life'. But changes were beginning to happen to my body—night sweats, low libido, periods of anxiety and depression, a few new hairy recruits to my face and sometimes irregular periods with clotting. I really knew nothing about this unspoken milestone in a woman's life. Was I supposed to dread the inevitable or rejoice in its arrival? I didn't have much information to go on. I certainly don't remember my mother having said a thing to me about her experience of menopause. It was as mysterious to me as my first initiation into womanhood— menstruation. At that time, I didn't know much about the workings of my body. And, in all honesty, I must admit that at forty-four years of age the physiology of the female body was still rather a mystery to me.

Thus, I began my exploration into the realm of menopause. I thought the exercise would be to simply learn the facts and, ultimately, to make an informed decision about Hormone Replacement Therapy. It turned out to be so much more. The curiosity which led me on this journey catapulted me into unexpected domains. Like Alice walking through the looking glass, I ventured into a topsy-turvy world where nothing was as it appeared to be. What was presented as truth upon closer scrutiny dissolved into illusion.

The more I explored this subject, the more I stumbled upon an entangled maze of myths, misinformation and propaganda. I discovered that the treatments of medical science for managing women's hormonal problems were fraught with many unseen dangers. While many of these treatments are proclaimed as either perfectly safe or having only minimal risks or side-effects, in actuality there is nothing safe about pharmaceutically or surgically tampering with women's hormones.

My continuing research caused me to challenge the most sacrosanct belief about the menopausal woman—that she is estrogen deficient. It was becoming apparent that 'estrogen deficiency' was a completely erroneous assumption. At first I could hardly believe what I was discovering. What about the millions of women around the world who are presently receiving synthetic hormones to correct their supposed 'estrogen deficiency'? Could it really be that all these women are being mis-diagnosed? Could it be that the medical profession, spurred on by the billion dollar pharmaceutical industry, was way off track? The simple answer is yes. The complex answer, however, requires delving much more deeply into a myriad of political, cultural and economic issues as well as conflicting paradigms.

As I sought out the researchers, medical doctors and writers who helped me to bring this picture into focus, the true story began to emerge. It involves not just the issue of menopause but the wide-scale use of synthetic estrogen and progestins (which is synthetic progesterone) to treat women at all ages of their life—from their teenage years right through to their post-menopausal years. The following chapters will provide a totally different perspective on the hormone story than has previously been available to most women and, for that matter, most health practitioners. I have written this book in simple language so that every woman (and man) can easily understand the issues at hand and the risks at stake.

But there is much more to this story. It involves a greater awareness of what is happening to our environment through the toxic estrogenic pollution from the indiscriminate use of herbicides, pesticides and plastics over the last two decades and the serious effects such changes have upon our hormonal health. It necessitates a reappraisal of our life-style—illustrating the importance and necessity of clean air, pure water and organic foods.

This story also concerns each woman's personal journey of empowerment and the honoring of her own intuitive wisdom. It's about women regaining responsibility for their own bodies and returning to a greater connection to natural cycles. Regaining this balance is crucial for the survival of our planet! It is, also intimately linked to finding the balance within oneself—physically, emotionally, mentally and spiritually.

As is so often the case, embarking upon this journey has

profoundly transformed me. My personal quest for most of my life has been to find within myself a deep sense of inner peace, confidence, self- acceptance and courage to express my creative gifts. It has been a long and often painful process with many recurring bouts of feeling inadequate and powerless.

Like so many other women, I was in a constant battle with my body, regularly assaulting it with diets, food fads, deprivation and disdain. These inner stresses would frequently manifest as allergies, irregular periods, fatigue, PMS, anxiety attacks and depression.

What began as curiosity about the changes occurring in my body gained momentum to become a quest for knowledge. Through the years I investigated natural alternatives to balance my hormones with dietary changes, herbs, meditation and exercise. Part of my personal quest was to reclaim my appreciation for being a woman. I realized that menstrual cycles expressed not only physical changes in my body but also psychological and spiritual changes—a part of the mystery of being female I never understood before. I began to listen more closely to my intuition and the needs of my body, emotions and spirit. I've now come to realize how truly miraculous it is to be a woman.

As I integrated this new awareness and these new behaviors, my life began to change. My body began to heal and eventually all my physical symptoms totally disappeared. Even those symptoms which I thought were the inevitable signs of menopause were more about the stress and disharmony within me than actual menopause. My health is now the best it has ever been. To my great delight I have also discovered a growing sense of well-being. I am no longer feeling afraid and insecure. As I continued to honor myself and my emotional and physical needs, I feel more centered within. I have at last arrived at a time of my life when I can honestly say I love who I am—a major accomplishment from those old days of self-hatred!

With each passing day I find myself tapping into to a more profound and personal understanding of feminine power. I have come to realize that for a woman to truly reclaim her true power, she must embody a deep appreciation and reverence for herself as an expression of the Feminine. It is a multi-faceted journey. Coming into hormonal balance requires a re-balancing and aligning on all levels. After all, our bodies are an expression of what we feed them—through our thoughts, our emotions, our diet, our actions and our creative expression. I have included in this book further information and practical strategies which I have personally experienced and from which I have benefited for creating this greater inner and outer balance.

By having the courage to explore, to question and even to challenge the status quo within myself as well as in the outer world, I am at last awakening to the power of my Feminine Self. Life is a most joyful and wondrous adventure for me now. And my wish is that as you read this book, you too will be inspired to begin your journey to greater health and feminine wisdom.

Hormone Heresy

Part One —

The Untold Hormone Story

Chapter 1

Getting the Story Straight

Synthetic hormones, in the form of estrogen or progestins, are quite high profile these days. For some they represent the Golden Fleece that excites so many medical practitioners, pharmaceutical companies and writers in search of their miraculous properties. For others, estrogen and progestin are rather perilous hormones, fraught with many unknown and unspoken dangers. Most women are lost in the dark and bottomless abyss, somewhere between truth and fiction. All to often they are desperately confused about whether to trust their instincts or medical science. Nothing less than their physical, emotional and mental health and long term well-being hang in the balance.

This hormone story is similar to a modern day thriller. It is a story of deception, betrayal, hidden agendas, propaganda and misinformation. As a story it could be quite entertaining but as a real life drama its effects are disastrous to the lives of tens of millions of women around the world.

Hormones are very powerful substances. Begin tampering with nature's finely tuned messengers of life's processes and you are asking for trouble. This is especially true for women. A woman's psyche is intimately connected to her monthly flow of hormones. Hormones not only direct and determine her physiological processes but also influence her emotional and psychological state. Besides creating a myriad of health problems and diseases, hormonal imbalance can undermine self-esteem, creativity, mental acuity and a healthy sex drive.

Perhaps the bigger picture about the hormone story lies in the fact that the introduction of synthetic hormones, as a purportedly legitimate need of women, is basically experimentation under the guise of standard medical practice. As a result, medical science has expanded its control over women's lives. A sense of powerlessness and hopelessness seem to permeate a woman's existence.

Germaine Greer, well-known feminist and author of *The Change*, sums up the medical establishment's intrusion into a woman's hormonal health quite astutely when she says, "Menopause is a dream speciality for the mediocre medic. It requires no surgical or diagnostic skill, it is not itself a life-threatening condition, there is no scope for malpractice action. Patients must return again and again for a battery of tests and check-ups."[1]

Quite simply, tampering with a woman's hormones is tampering with her power.

The Waning of Women's Health and Power

For over three hundred years, beginning in the thirteenth century and continuing well into the sixteenth century, the Inquisition was a reign of terror to the vast majority of peoples living throughout Europe and Scandinavia. The political, economic and religious forces of that time joined together to consolidate their power by eliminating those whom they perceived as impeding their ultimate objectives.

The unfortunate target of their efforts were the keepers of the healing arts and the ancient spiritual and cultural wisdom. Historians debate the exact toll of such a hellish time—whether it was several hundreds of thousands or as many as nine million—but what is undebatable is that the vast majority of victims were women. In fact, the Inquisition is now regarded as a period of genocide against women which successfully divested them of their power, self-respect, wealth, healing arts, prominence and influence in their communities.

The Inquisition guaranteed that the Church fathers were the undisputable spiritual authorities. It was also successful in enshrining medical knowledge securely in the realm of men since the Inquisition decreed that only trained medical doctors could now practice the healing arts. Needless to say, medical schools were barred to women (so, for that matter, was any formal education).

What a relief that such a violent and misogynist era ended long ago. Or did it? Unfortunately, it appears that some traditions linger on. Women of today are still prey to vast political and economic interests, suffering dire consequences to their health, financial independence and personal power. Perhaps the Inquisition hasn't ended at all, but merely taken a more subtle and devious form.

Certainly an astute observation was made by Sandra Coney in her book, *The Menopause Industry*, where she says, "the mid-life woman is oblivious to the deeply sexist ideology underlying the options she has laid down before her. Naively she may think these are offered simply for her own benefit. She is not cognizant of the others who benefit or may also be served by her decisions. She is unaware, too, that the options themselves may be incompletely tested, that there may be considerable controversy about them in the medical literature and that doctors will differ in their views. What she is told—how much or how little—is mediated by her doctor. The end result is a woman poorly placed to decide for herself."

The influence of the medical and pharmaceutical interests exert on women is overwhelming. And it's no wonder. The fact is that women are very big business.The lucrative market spans all age groups of women from young teenagers to the postmenopausal. Synthetic hormones, surgical procedures, drugs, medical tests, diagnostic tests and on-going doctor's visits (not to mention the complications incurred from all of these) makes gynecology a most lucrative speciality.

Since the introduction of the Pill, 200 million women around the world have taken it. In the United States alone, 50 million women have used oral contraceptives. In 1988, an estimated 10 million women were on them.

Hysterectomies are another big industry. The Pill has been a significant contributor to conditions that later on necessitate the removal of a woman's uterus and ovaries. To date it has been estimated that 20 million women have had their uteruses removed. Close to one million American women have hysterectomies each year. Of those women, 42 percent of the time they will also have their ovaries removed. It's shocking to realize that presently 1 out of 3 women in the U.S. will have a hysterectomy by 60 years of age. What's even more shocking is that three quarters of the hysterectomies performed are on women under the age of 49. Removal of the uterus as well as the ovaries will immediately catapult a women into "surgical menopause" which necessitates hormones. What's more an oophorectomy (removal of the ovaries), medically classified as a castration, will also require more hormones.

By the year 2000, fifty million American women will be entering menopause. Presently 15 to 30 percent of the country's

40 million menopausal or postmenopausal women have been prescribed synthetic hormones. As the number of conditions that are conjured up that supposedly benefit from HRT such as cardiovascular disease, osteoporosis and Alzheimer's disease grow in number, the net covering the female population widens even more.

The total cost from these chemical and surgical procedures is astronomical - billions upon billions of dollars. The estrogen drug, Premarin, which is presently the most widely prescribed drug in the U.S. alone grosses approximately $940 million dollars a year. That's just one drug! The hysterectomy industry is reputed to be worth more than 4 billion dollars. So it's no wonder that the medical industry views women as an unlimited resource to be plundered. When it comes to profits, unbiased controlled studies, long-term trials as well as natural alternatives are all sacrificed for the insatiable hunger for profits.

Nor is it an accident that gynecologists happen to be one of the highest earners of all specialists and that throughout a woman's life she is encouraged to be continuously medicalized. Natural female functions from menstruation through childbirth and then on into menopause are taken over by medical and pharmaceutical interventions. Barraged by a litany of false claims, emotive advertising campaigns, and, in some cases, downright lies, it's no wonder that so many women are thoroughly confused about matters relating to the health of their own bodies.

The History of Hormone Replacement

Perhaps there is no topic of greater confusion to women than the highly publicized introduction of Hormone Replacement Therapy for the menopausal woman. It has been receiving tremendous attention in our culture as the Baby Boomers come of menopausal age. It is touted as the best thing for liberating women since the discovery of oral contraceptives (even though the statistics now show that wide use of the Pill has given rise to health hazards such as breast cancer, high blood pressure and cardiovascular disease on a scale previously unknown in medicine).[3]

Investigation into the theory of hormone replacement goes all the way back to the 1930's with the research of Dr. Serge Voronoff. His research involved implanting fresh monkeys testicles into men's scrotums with limited effectiveness. Offshoots of his research led to the grafting of monkey ovaries into women with rather dire consequences. After several fatalities (to both monkeys and women), the search was redirected to the use of synthetic estrogen. With the onset of World War II things were put on hold.

Menopause didn't really come into vogue as a topic of concern for the medical profession until the 1960's. In 1966 a New York gynecologist, Dr. Robert Wilson, wrote a best seller called *Feminine Forever*, extolling the virtues of estrogen replacement to save women from the "tragedy of menopause which often destroys her character as well as her health." Feeding upon women's greatest fears, his book sold over 100,000 copies the first year. Wilson energetically promoted menopause as a condition of 'living decay'. According to him, estrogen replacement was a kind of long sought after youth pill that would save poor fading women from the horrors of age.

He popularized the erroneous belief that menopause was a deficiency disease.

Some of the myths which his book helped to enshrine amongst the general population as well as the medical community included:

... Ovaries shrivel up and die as a result of menopause.

... The woman becomes the equivalent of a eunuch.

... I have known cases where the resulting physical and mental anguish was so unbearable that the patient committed suicide.

... I have seen untreated women who had shriveled into caricatures of their former selves.

... Though the physical suffering from menopausal effects can be truly dreadful, what impressed me the most tragically is the destruction of the personality.

... To be desexed is to her a staggering catastrophe.

... She is incapable of rationally perceiving her own situation.

... The transformation within a few years of a formerly pleasant, energetic woman into a dull-minded but sharp-tongued caricature of her former self is one of the saddest of human spectacles.

... In a maze of longing and delusion they sometimes lose touch with reality and thus a menopausal neurosis develops.

Women's magazines eagerly seized upon his ideas and extensively promoted his concepts. This pleased Wilson immensely, having earlier set up the Wilson Foundation for the sole purpose of promoting the use of estrogen drugs.

The pharmaceutical industry generously contributed over 1.3 million dollars to his Foundation. Each year he received funds from companies such as Searle, Wyeth-Ayerst Laboratories and Upjohn which made hormone products that Wilson claimed were effective in treating and preventing menopause.[4] Pharmaceutical companies jumped on the bandwagon with aggressive promotions and advertising campaigns. His message hit a receptive chord—mid-life women need hormone drugs to be rescued from the inevitable horrors and decrepitude of this terrible deficiency disease called menopause.

Wilson pioneered the use of 'unopposed estrogen' which is synthetic estrogen prescribed on its own. However, there had been no formal assessment of the safety of estrogen therapy or its long term effects. Unopposed estrogen went out of vogue when it became very apparent that it shortened the life-span of its users. In 1975, the *New England Journal of Medicine* examined the rates of endometrial cancer for estrogen consumers concluding that the risk was seven-and-a-half times greater for estrogen users. Women who had used estrogen for seven years or longer were 14 times more likely to develop cancer.[5] Wilson's theories then fell out of favor and the FDA told the drug companies that he was an "unacceptable investigator".

As the popularity of unopposed estrogen therapy waned, new approaches were sought. The focus was directed away from the false claims of preserving feminine beauty and youthfulness to relieving menopausal symptoms. The pharmaceutical industry resurrected Estrogen Replacement Therapy in the form of the new 'safe' Hormone Replacement Therapy, a combination of synthetic progesterone (progestin) and estrogen. HRT would supposedly protect menopausal women not only from cardiovascular disease, but also the ravages of osteoporosis. The latest contentious discovery is estrogen's part in preventing Alzheimers.

Another Perspective

While the so-called 'experts' on women's health are reassuring women that there are only very minor and insignificant side-effects, Dr. Lynette J. Dumble, Senior Research Fellow at the University of Melbourne in Australia, believes, "the sole basis of HRT is to create a commercial market that is highly profitable for the pharmaceutical companies and doctors. The supposed benefits of HRT are totally unproven." She believes that HRT not only exacerbates a woman's health problems but contributes to the acceleration of her aging process. HRT either hastens the onset of other medical conditions or worsens existing ones.

This perspective seems to be validated by the most recent findings from the National Institute of Health's sponsored *Boston Nurses Questionnaire Study* that followed 121,700 women for the past 18 years. The study revealed startling effects from HRT. It warned that women who used the combined progestin and estrogen of HRT increased their chances of developing breast cancer by up to 100 percent if taking the hormone for ten years or more. The study found ten years of use of estrogen alone increased the risk of breast cancer by 30-40 percent compared with women of the same age who never used postmenopausal HRT. Thus revealing that the combination of estrogen and progestin was risky business when it comes to breast cancer.

But even only five years of use has its dangers. The risk increased 30-40 percent if HRT is used five or more years. In women aged between 60-64 years the risk of breast cancer rose to 70 percent after five years of HRT. Finally, the study concluded that women using HRT were 45 percent more likely to die from breast cancer than those who chose not to use HRT or used it for less than five years.[6]

Dr. Graham Colditz, the study's principal researcher from Harvard recommends that women should only use HRT for relief of menopausal symptoms and for no longer than two or three years.

According to Leslie Kenton, the author of *Passage to Power*, "Everybody who is anybody will tell you that menopause is an estrogen deficiency disease and that you will need to take more estrogen as you approach mid-life. What may surprise you is this: not only is most of such commonly given advice on menopause wrong, a great deal of it can be positively dangerous."

Similar in his view of menopause is Dr. John Lee, retired physician and author of *What Doctors May Not Tell You About Menopause*. "Menopause per se should be regarded as a normal adjustment reflecting a benign change in a woman's biological life away from child bearing and onward to a period of new personal power and fulfillment. The western perception of menopause as a threshold of undesirable symptoms and regressive illness due to estrogen deficiency is an error not supported by fact. More accurately, we should view our menopause problem as an abnormality brought about by industrialized cultures' deviation from a healthy life-style." The June 1996 *Townsend Letter for Doctors and Patients* points out that dietary, exercise and life-style factors have been shown to offer identical benefits to the proclaimed benefits of HRT without the risks.

It is becoming quite evident that there is another side to the Hormone Story—a perspective that can assist women of all ages to attain greater health and reclaim a greater sense of power, responsibility and dignity in their lives.

Chapter 2

A Brief Gynecological Tour of a Woman's Body

In order to understand the HRT debate and for that matter, the whole synthetic hormone issue, it is important to first have a rudimentary knowledge of a woman's body and its cyclic nature. As educated as we are as women, there seems to be a huge gap when it comes to having a meaningful and accurate understanding of the most intimate aspect of ourselves—our body.

Until recently doctors thought that menopause began when all the eggs in the ovaries had been used up. However, later work has shown that menopause is probably not triggered by the ovaries but by the brain. It seems that both puberty and menopause are brain-driven events.

So let us begin upon a fundamental understanding of the physiology of the female body.

The ovaries, located at either side of the uterus, are the primary sex organs. They are about 1 1/4 inches long and are shaped like prunes. At birth they contain all of the immature eggs, also known as follicles, that will mature and be released during a woman's fertile life. The developing fetus contains about seven million follicles; at birth the number of follicles are reduced to about two million. By the time puberty arrives there exists about 400,000 follicles, although only about 400 of them actually develop during a woman's fertile lifetime.

A follicle is a balloon-like sac which holds the immature egg in a protective fluid. As the egg follicles grow, they manufacture and release estrogen (estradiol) into the blood. After ten or twelve days, one of the developing egg cells out of the six to twenty that develop during a menstrual cycle moves to the outer surface of the ovary. The follicle then ejects the egg into the abdominal cavity where it finds its way into the fallopian tube for slow transportation to the uterus.

A normal menstrual cycle of every 26 to 28 days depends on a complex network of hormonal communications between the ovaries, the hypothalamus and the pituitary gland in the brain. All the hormones released are secreted not in a constant, steady way but at dramatically different rates during the 28 day menstrual cycle.

The development of the immature egg is initiated by the brain-controlled hypothalamus through a sex-gland-stimulating hormone called gonadotropin-releasing hormone (GrRH). GrRH then stimulates the pituitary to release two more substances into the blood stream. These two hormones are called follicle stimulating hormone (FSH) and luteinizing hormone (LH). Throughout the month, a constant feedback loop creates a continuous adjustment and regulation of the hormone levels between the brain and the ovaries.

On cue from FSH, estrogen triggers an egg to begin ripening, stimulates the buildup of tissue and blood in the uterus and controls the first part of the cycle. Estrogen production gradually builds to a peak just before ovulation, then levels off for the remainder of the cycle, dropping again to low amounts at menstruation.

Estrogen also generates the changes that take place at puberty—the growth of breasts, the development of the reproductive system and the shape of a woman's body. Around the time of ovulation, estrogen also causes changes in the vaginal mucus, making it more tolerant of male penetration during sexual activity and more hospitable to sperm. As estrogen levels rise and ovulation is approached, the mucus becomes more profuse, thinner, wetter and clearer. At this time, just before ovulation and as estrogen peaks, the mucus becomes jelly-like, resembling raw egg white, and can be stretched between the fingers. This is a signal that ovulation is imminent. This period of time from the beginning of menstruation until the onset of ovulation is called the follicular stage .

On the other hand, prompted by LH, the ovaries dramatically increase their output of progesterone at the time of ovulation, about twelve to thirteen days into the cycle. Progesterone production during this phase of the cycle, called the luteal phase, leads to a refinement and 'ripening' of tissue and blood in the uterus. Progesterone also contributes to the changes in the vaginal mucus at the time of ovulation. The rise of progesterone at ovulation causes a rise in body temperature of about one degree Fahrenheit, a measure often used as one of the indications of ovulation.

Progesterone also plays a part in the mystery of the functioning of the follicles. Betty Kamen, Ph.D. author of *Hormone Replacement: Yes or No,* describes this process, "Follicles also communicate chemically with each other through a mechanism not yet fully understood. Only one follicle in one ovary continues to develop throughout the cycle. The egg-producing ovary sends a message to the other ovary to refrain from doing the same. The presence of progesterone initiates this "cease and desist" order. The growth of the chosen follicle continues to accelerate. During the last two days before ovulation, this follicle may be as large as three-quarters of an inch!"[1]

Immediately upon release of the egg on day fourteen, the fully matured follicle promoted by LH now functions in a different way. One of the wonders of the female body is the

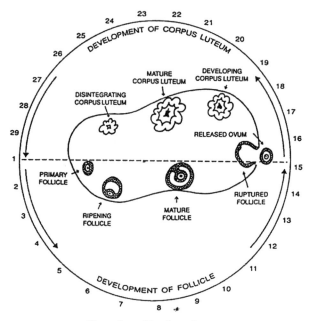

Ovarian Cycle - figure 1.

transformation of a follicle, upon release of the egg, into an endocrine gland called the corpus luteum which appears as a blister on the surface of the ovary. It is named corpus luteum because of its appearance as a small yellow, glandular mass. While it still continues to produce estrogen, it also becomes the prime production site of progesterone which dominates the second half of the menstrual cycle. When progesterone peaks, there is about 140 times as much progesterone as estrogen.

What is rarely understood is that the heightened sexual energy many women experience at the time of ovulation is the result of the surge of progesterone levels at the time of ovulation. Progesterone is the hormone necessary for increased libido, not estrogen as is commonly believed.

As the egg is ripening in the ovary, the uterus is ripening in preparation for the possibility of a growing fetus. The uterine lining thickens and becomes engorged with blood that will nourish a growing embryo. If no fertilized egg implants itself in the uterus, it then sheds its lining. This shedding is the blood of menstruation. Then the cycle begins again with the signal from the brain telling the ovary to begin ripening another egg.

According to Dr. Susan Love, author of *Dr. Susan Loves's Hormone Book*, "It can take a while for this dance of hormones to get its choreography down. One study confirmed that earlier on, girls have longer periods. The follicles don't mature, and there may be a longer time between periods. This seems to be in part because the ovaries aren't yet really producing eggs and egg production is necessary for a regular "loop" to be completed. Once the whole system gets coordinated, a girl's cycles become regular and her symptoms settle down."[2]

If pregnancy occurs, progesterone production increases and the shedding of the lining of the uterus is prevented, thus preserving the developing embryo. As pregnancy progresses, progesterone production is taken over by the placenta and its secretion increases gradually to levels of 300 to 400 milligrams during the third trimester. It is also associated with the increased sense of well-being that women feel at this stage of their pregnancy.

As was previously mentioned, ovarian estrogen and progesterone stimulate the growth of the lining of the uterus in preparation for fertilization. Estrogen proliferates the growth of endometrium tissue and progesterone facilitates its further maturing so the fertilized egg can implant successfully. Adequate progesterone, therefore, is the hormone most essential to the survival of the fertilized egg and the fetus. It appears that the lack of adequate levels of progesterone at this time contributes to difficulties in conception and a high

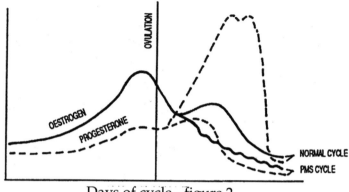

Days of cycle - figure 2.

risk of miscarriage.

At around 40 years of age, the interaction between hormones alters, eventually leading to menopause. It is still not clear how. Menopause may start with changes in the hypothalamus and the pituitary gland rather than the ovary. Scientists have conducted experiments where young mice have their ovaries replaced with those from aged animals that are no longer capable of reproducing. The results showed that they were then able to mate and give birth. This shows that an old ovary placed in a young environment is capable of responding. On the other hand, when young ovaries were put into old mice, they were not able to reproduce.

Whatever the mechanism triggering menopause, as fewer egg follicles are stimulated, the amount of estrogen and progesterone being produced by the ovaries decline, although the other hormones continue to be produced. Estrogen levels drop to only 40-60 percent at menopause, just low enough so that follicles do not mature, thus making pregnancy impossible. Contrary to popular belief, the ovaries do not shrivel up nor do they cease functioning. With the reduction of these hormones, menstruation becomes scantier and erratic and finally ceases.

Doctors who see the ovaries as useless after menopause point out that in women's older years the ovaries grow smaller. However, as women age, part of the ovary that shrinks is known as the theca, the outermost covering where the eggs grow and develop. The innermost part of the ovary, known as the inner stoma, actually becomes active at menopause for the first time in a woman's life. With exquisite timing, one function starts up as the other winds down.

After menopause the ovaries continue to function working in conjunction with other body sites such as the adrenal glands, skin, muscle, brain, pineal gland, hair follicles and body fat to produce hormones. Celso Ramon Garcia, M.D., Director Of Surgery at the Hospital of the University of Pennsylvania, is one of the many authorities saying that the hormones produced by the postmenopausal ovaries promote bone health and skin suppleness, support sexual functioning, protect against heart disease and contribute to a woman's health and well-being.

The uterus is another misunderstood and denigrated organ by a medical profession which continues to reassure women that uteruses are disposable organs that they can quite happily live without. Women are thus encouraged to embrace hysterectomies as a salvation to so many of their "female problems". *The People's Doctor Newsletter*, (Oct 1989) report that what few women are aware of is that far from being a useless and unnecessary organ once a woman's childbearing days are over, the uterus is actually the main site for the production of the hormone prostacyclin which protects women from heart disease and unwanted blood-clotting. Since prostacyclin

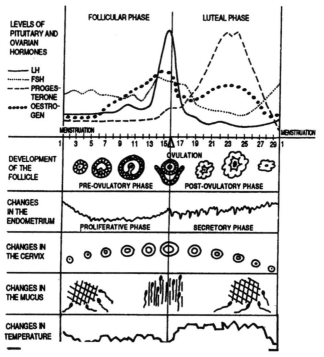

Female hormone levels during a monthly cycle - figure 3.

cannot be manufactured in a laboratory, the removal of the uterus will ensure its production will cease forever.

Provided a woman has taken good care of herself during the peri-menopausal years with proper life-style, diet and mental and emotional health, the female body is quite capable of making healthy adjustments in hormonal balance after menopause.

Menopausal women have the opportunity to enter this phase of life empowered in their wisdom and creativity as never before. They have access to profound inner knowing.

The renowned sociologist, Margaret Mead, stated the now

famous decree, "There is nothing more powerful than a meno-pausal woman with zest!" In many cultures around the world, menopause is a transition and an initiation into the fulfillment of a woman's power—totally symptom-free. She is held in the highest regard in her community as a wise, respected elder.

Unfortunately, as we will explore this natural adjustment of hormonal levels designed by nature to be a gradual and undramatic transition has been seriously altered for many women throughout the industrialized world.

Chapter 3

The Myth of Synthetic Estrogen and Progestins

The earlier research that led to the synthesis of estrogen made possible the development of the oral contraceptive in 1960. With the consent of the US Food and Drug Administration (FDA), the Pill was widely marketed as an effective, convenient method of birth control. True sexual liberation for women was at hand at last—or so we thought.

However, the entire basis for the FDA's consent was the result of clinical studies conducted on 132 Puerto Rican women who had taken the Pill for one year or longer. (However, there were five women who died during the study without any investigation into the cause of their deaths.)[1]

By the mid-1970's the death toll of women from heart attacks and strokes began to attract public notice. A newer, supposedly safer Pill was then created with a lower dose of estrogen. In fact, there has never been any valid scientific proof that the Pill was safe nor, for that matter, were any of the other forms of contraception presently available. Women are only now discovering the price they have been paying for their sexual freedom. By altering their hormonal balance, many varied and devastating emotional and physiological dysfunctions have been created.

It is now almost 40 years since the first introduction of oral contraception and there are presently about 60 million women worldwide who are, in effect, 'trialing' the Pill. Its safety and long-term effects have still not been conclusively established. It is interesting to note, however, that the Pill has produced a wide assortment of adverse effects and significant links have been established to breast cancer, high blood pressure and, in particular, cardiovascular disease, the major cause of female deaths.

Over 180,000 U.S. women are diagnosed with breast cancer every year and 46,000 deaths occur. Breast cancer incidence has gone up three percent a year every year since 1980. In 1940, a woman's life time risk of breast cancer was 1 in 16; that figure has now risen to 1 in 8.[1] Is this merely a coincidence or do these statistics indicate, perhaps, the harmful side effects of interfering with hormones?

While proclaimed as the primary missing ingredient for the menopausal woman, estrogen is also strongly recommended by the medical and pharmaceutical industries for the prevention of cardiovascular disease and osteoporosis. It is available in a variety of forms—pills, patches and implants. These days, most doctors will warn women of the inherent risks of going through menopause and, for that matter, the post-menopausal years without the essential protection of estrogen. Women are further reminded that menopause is a deficiency disease which supposedly means they are lacking estrogen and therefore must have supplemental doses to insure their health is maintained.

As Dr. Lynette Dumble has noted, "Broadly speaking, cardiovascular prevention in women has overwhelmingly focused on hormone replacement. Yet, as Elizabeth Barrett-Connor emphasizes, *The Big Trial*, the Coronary Drug Project of 1973 that included two estrogen regimens, was conducted on men. As part of *The Big Trial* design, estrogen doses extravagantly in excess of physiological levels were deliberately administered to men in order to induce gynecomastia (enlargement of male breasts) as an indication of successful feminization. This resulted in thrombosis and impotence and ultimately led to research failure because of treatment discontinuation amongst the study's participants."[2]

According to Dr. John Lee, the one notable study which formed the entire basis of the positive estrogen-cardiovascular link, known as the *Boston Nurses Questionnaire Study* and conducted with a large sampling of nurses, was radically flawed. Although there is ample evidence from numerous other studies showing that, indeed, the opposite is true—estrogen is a significant factor in creating heart disease—these findings have been virtually ignored in the frenzy for profits. He goes on to say that the pharmaceutical advertisements also neglected to mention the fact that stroke death incidence from that study was 50 percent higher among the estrogen users.

Dr. Lee has compiled a list of side-effects and physiological impairment which occurs from taking estrogen. These include increased risk of endometrial cancer, increased body fat, salt and fluid retention, depression and headaches, impaired blood sugar control (hypoglycemia), loss of zinc and retention of copper, reduced oxygen levels in all cells, thickened bile and gall bladder disease, increased likelihood of breast fibrocysts and uterine fibroids. Estrogen replacement interfered with thyroid activity, decreased sex drive, caused excessive blood clotting, reduced vascular tone and caused endometriosis, uterine cramping, infertility and restraint of osteoclast function.

With so many side-effects and dangerous complications, a woman must think very carefully about the HRT decision. Unfortunately, most doctors will say there is no other alternative and that it is relatively safe. While certainly most doctors are well meaning and sincerely concerned about their patients, their primary source of education and product information comes directly from the pharmaceutical companies. Since most women also lack essential education and understanding about their options, menopause can be perceived as a rather frightening and perilous time. Women fear that if they don't follow their doctor's advice (after all he really does know best), then they may face the remaining years of their life with the threat of great suffering and physical deterioration. Women are often in for a rude awakening when they experience firsthand, just how badly their health needs have been managed.

Chapter 4

A Lesson From History

One of the greatest gifts of history is the ability to assess past events and past actions so that we can learn from our mistakes. The wisdom of hindsight can greatly assist us in making more appropriate choices to guide us safely into the future. Unfortunately, we rarely learn from the past and seem to be doomed to repeating our mistakes. When it comes to the widespread and indiscriminate use of synthetic hormones, there are many powerful lessons to draw upon.

One of the most poignant and tragic stories of synthetic hormones gone tragically wrong occurred with the introduction of a drug called diethylstilbestrol (DES for short), a synthetic estrogen prescribed to many pregnant women in the mistaken belief that it prevented miscarriage and pregnancy complications. The drug was widely prescribed for between four and six million pregnant women in the United States and Europe. Estimates in the US put DES exposure at between 2.7 and 5.4 percent of the total US population in 1979.

The DES story illustrates the failure of the medical profession, health authorities and drug companies to report the dangers, acknowledge the warnings and then take action to protect the public. This is also the story of a time-bomb still ticking away, not only in the innocent women who were administered the drug, but also in their daughters and sons with potential repercussions for generations to come.

Dishonest Beginnings

The story begins in the early 1940's, when Drs. George and Olive Smith, a husband and wife team from the Harvard Medical School, began theorizing about the use of a new drug, DES, in maintaining high-risk pregnancies. The maternity hospital associated with Harvard was used by the Smith's to test their theories.

Although DES was proved toxic in several early animal tests, these were largely ignored and DES was eventually marketed with the blessings of the FDA as a safe and effective drug to prevent miscarriage.

Dr. Robin Rowland, in her book, *Living Laboratories*, pointed out that "some of the women given this drug were used as experimental subjects and were told that they were taking a vitamin tablet". [1]

As the word spread throughout the medical community, DES was also prescribed as an estrogen replacement in menopause, as a 'morning after' pill (actually a five day treatment), to suppress lactation, as a treatment for acne, to treat certain types of breast and prostate cancer and to inhibit growth in young girls. It was primarily given in tablet form, but could also be injected or implanted. For several decades there was an additional use for DES. It was added to cattle feed as a 'growth promoter'.

The reason that DES has been likened to a time-bomb is that the drug companies assured the doctors that DES was perfectly safe. It has taken many years for the serious long-term effects of DES on the women themselves, as well as to their daughters and sons, to be revealed. And the story isn't over yet.

The Truth Comes to Light

In 1984, the first major study of breast cancer risks for DES mothers was published in the *New England Journal of Medicine*. It reported that some twenty years after taking DES, mothers had a 40 to 50 percent greater risk than non-exposed mothers.[2]

More shocking realizations about the indiscriminate use of DES during pregnancy surfaced in the early 1970's. What had, up until then, been an exceptionally rare form of vaginal cancer occurring in women after menopause suddenly began appearing in young women (in all the world's prior medical literature there were only three cases reported developing in young women). Mysteriously, within a short period of time eight women were admitted to a Boston hospital diagnosed with this rare vaginal cancer. Their cancers were all traced back to the DES given to their mothers in pregnancy some 20 years earlier. Presently over 600 cases have been reported.

Since these initial ominous revelations, more effects of DES have emerged and been reported in medical journals. They include:[3]

1. Many DES daughters have benign tissue and structural damage to the vagina and cervix relating to their DES exposure.

2. Abnormalities of the uterus and fallopian tubes have been found, the common and characteristic change being a T-shaped uterus with a small uterine cavity. These abnormalities are suspected as possible causative factors in the higher incidence of pregnancy difficulties.

3. DES daughters, when compared with a non-exposed control group, experienced 3 to 5 times the rate of ectopic pregnancy; at least twice the rate of miscarriage in the first and second trimester; and at least three times the rate of pre mature labor, premature birth or stillbirth. It appears that as many as 50 percent of DES daughters will experience these reproductive complications.

4. Recent research findings have revealed that DES daughters have between a two and four-fold increased incidence of squamous cell dysplasia and cervical cancer. This possibility was suggested over a decade ago, following experiments with animals.

5. Approximately one third of DES sons have structural abnormalities of the genital tract including a history of undescended testicles (a known risk factor for contracting testicular cancer), cysts and lowered sperm counts. Some sons may be infertile.

6. DES exposure can also result in an impaired immune system. Certain conditions, including respiratory tract infections, asthma, arthritis and lupus were reported more frequently among the DES-exposed men and women.

What will happen to the DES daughters as they approach menopause? We won't have to wait too long before the answer becomes apparent.

At the 10th International Congress of Psychosomatic Obstetrics and Gynecology held in Stockholm in June 1992, various speakers gave the chilling news that to this day certain manufacturers of DES, unable to sell this drug in Western nations for use in pregnancy, are successfully promoting and selling it throughout the third world! How much more human misery will the drug companies be responsible for?

All the warning signals are there. When it comes to the enthusiastic prescribing of synthetic hormones either in the form of estrogen, progestin or any others, are we doomed to repeat history as we once again interfere with women's natural hormonal production?

DES Support Group

DES Action USA
1615 Broadway - Suite 510
Oakland, California 94612
Tel: 1-800-DES-9288 or (510) 465 4011 Fax: (510) 465 4815
Internet desact@well.sf.ca.us

Chapter 5

Introducing Estrogen Dominance

The natural design of the body is to produce the two hormones, progesterone and estrogen, in a very sensitive and precise balance so that reproductive ability is maximized. These two hormones are closely interrelated in many ways and although they are generally antagonistic towards each other, each helps the other by making the cells of a target organ more sensitive.

Estrogen isn't really a single hormone. 'Estrogen' refers to a class of hormones with estrus activity (i.e., proliferation of endometrial cells in preparation for pregnancy). These estrogens include estradiol and estrone, both of which are implicated in stimulating abnormal cell growth when found in higher than normal amounts in the body, and estriol which is known to be cancer inhibiting. Each type of estrogen has a different function in the body. These estrogens are produced mainly in the ovaries, although small quantities are secreted from the adrenal glands, the placenta during pregnancy and fat cells.

At puberty, estrogen in a girl encourages the development of breasts and the expansion of the uterus. Estrogen contributes to the moulding of female body contours and maturation of the skeleton. After that, estrogens help regulate the menstrual cycle and plays other necessary roles to maintain bone mass and keep blood cholesterol levels in check.

When excessive quantities of estrogens, regardless of source, are present in a young woman's body they will contribute to the 'burn out' of her ovaries and undermine fertility.

In the case of progesterone, however, we are talking about one specific hormone. Thus, progesterone is both the name of the class and the single member of the class. In the ovaries, progesterone is the precursor of estrogen. Progesterone is also made in smaller amounts by the adrenal glands in both sexes and by the testes in males. It is also the precursor of testosterone and all important adrenocortical hormones. In addition to the sex hormones, corticosteroids are also derived from progesterone. Corticosteroids are essential for stress response, sugar and electrolyte balance and blood pressure, not to mention survival.[1]

While estrogen is the primary hormone during the first two weeks of a woman's menstrual cycle, fulfilling its role of preparing the endometrium for pregnancy, progesterone is the major female reproductive hormone during the latter two weeks of the menstrual cycle. Progesterone is necessary for the survival of the fertilized ovum, the resulting embryo and the fetus throughout gestation when production of the progesterone is taken over by the placenta.

One of the functions of estrogen is to store the energy derived from food as fat. This is why estrogen is readily given to cattle. Since cattle are sold by body weight, the more they're fattened up the more they're worth. Estrogen also adds weight by increasing water retention. It's no wonder estrogen has been so widely used in the meat industry (and a good reason to avoid all meat products that are not organically raised). Progesterone, on the other hand, turns fat into energy. Increasing progesterone levels contributes to weight loss and higher levels of energy.

There is a very delicate balance between the interplay of estrogen and progesterone. If that balance is interfered with, devastating effects occur. Unfortunately, introduced synthetic hormones, as well as environmental pollutants, are presently wreaking havoc with our hormones.

Growing Hormonal Imbalances

'Estrogen Dominance' is a term that was first used by Dr. John Lee. For the better part of the last two decades, Dr. Lee has been exploring the basis for the proliferation of such female problems as PMS, endometriosis, ovarian cysts, fibroids, breast cancer, infertility, osteoporosis and menopausal problems. From his clinical experience in the field of female health and from his published research, Dr. Lee believes that many women are suffering from the effects of too much estrogen. He finds that stress, nutritional deficiencies, estrogenic substances from our environment and taking synthetic estrogens combined with an ensuing deficiency of progesterone are the likely contributing factors to the creation of estrogen dominance.

Dr. Lee has discovered a consistent theme running through women's complaints about the distressing and often debilitating symptoms of PMS, peri-menopause and menopause—too much estrogen, or estrogen dominance. Now, instead of estrogen playing its essential role within the well balanced symphony of steroid hormones in a woman's body, it has begun to overshadow the other players, creating biochemical dissonance. The last thing a woman's body needs is more estrogen—either in the form of contraceptives or HRT. And when estrogen dominance symptoms appear, guess what is prescribed? Even more estrogen! The delicate natural estrogen/progesterone balance is radically altered due to this excess of estrogen. Progesterone deficiency is then exacerbated.

Some of the side-effects of unopposed estrogen include an influx of water and sodium into the cells, thus affecting aldosterone production, leading to water retention and hypertension. Estrogen causes intracellular hypoxia (oxygen deprivation), opposes the action of the thyroid, promotes histamine release, promotes blood clotting thus increasing the risk of strokes and embolisms. Estrogen unopposed by progesterone also decreases libido, increases the likelihood of breast fibrocysts, uterine fibroids, uterine (endometrial) cancer and breast cancer.[2]

Female Health Problems on the Rise

Female problems seem to be on the rise. Between 40 and 60 percent of all women in the western societies suffer from Premenstrual Syndrome (PMS). In addition, women can suffer from a whole plethora of symptoms—some menopausal and others not. Something quite alarming certainly seems to be happening to women. There are indications that the proper hormonal balance necessary for a woman's body to function healthily is being seriously interfered with by a number of factors.

When a healthy woman has her menstrual flow, it is the time of her cycle when she is making essentially very little, of either hormone. Estrogen production begins to increase about eight days after her period has started. Normally, from day 12 to day 26, there are hundreds of times more progesterone being produced than estrogen. So, if progesterone is missing, estrogen is then circulating continuously from day 8 to day 26. Essentially, if a woman has a whole month of nothing but estrogen, that woman will be estrogen dominant.

Research has revealed that a good portion of women in their 30's (some even younger)—long before menopause—will, on occasion, not ovulate during their menstrual cycle. Even though they still menstruate, they are not producing an egg. Without ovulation, no corpus luteum results and no progesterone is able to be made. This is called an anovulatory cycle. A progesterone deficiency will then ensue. The frequency of these anovulatory cycles increases as menopause approaches, changing the menstrual pattern to either a heavier or longer menstrual flow.

Several serious problems can result from anovulatory cycles. This will cause her to have menopausal symptoms such as weight gain, water retention and mood swings. It used to be true that the majority of women began menopause in their mid forties or early fifties. In the last generation, however, it appears that the pattern is changing. It is now becoming more frequent for women to be experiencing anovulatory periods in their early thirties without the cessation of periods (menopause) until their late fifties. Therefore, these women have a month-long presence of unopposed estrogen in their bodies with all the attendant side effects.

A progesterone deficiency can also seriously affect bones and is of great concern in the development of osteoporosis. Contemporary medicine is still largely unaware that progesterone stimulates osteoblast-mediated new bone formation. What that means is that progesterone actually stimulates the growth of new bone tissue and therefore osteoporosis can be reversed at any age. Lack of progesterone means that new osteoblasts are not created, potentially giving rise to osteoporosis.[3]

A third major problem results from the inter-relationship between loss of progesterone and stress. When under stress, progesterone is converted into cortisol, the " fight or flight" hormone, at the expense of progesterone and estrogen. Stress combined with an unhealthy diet can induce anovulatory cycles. The consequent lack of progesterone interferes with the production of stress-combating hormones, thus exacerbating stressful conditions that give rise to further anovulatory cycles. Stress, nutritional deficiencies and chemical pollutants can all contribute to anovulatory cycles. And so the vicious cycle of progesterone deficiency continues.

It is important to note that, while the problem is recognized as a progesterone deficiency, it is not always true that progesterone levels are lower than normal but they may be low in comparison to elevated estrogen levels. Nevertheless, the delicate balance between estrogen and progesterone is significantly impaired. While not commonly understood by medical science, the growing incidence of anovulatory cycles, even in young women and the ensuing hormone imbalance is creating huge health problems. Women of all ages are now at higher risk of the entire range of estrogen dominant conditions. According to Dr. Lee, many of these common health problems can be offset by increasing the level of natural progesterone in the body.

Peri-menopause

Menopause is not a sudden or unexpected event that occurs to a woman one day but rather a gradual process that may begin for her about ten years prior to the cessation of her periods, anywhere from the ages of thirty five through to her late forties. There are many factors that contribute to the hormonal changes occurring in her body. They include heredity, environment, life-style, the age at which she first menstruated, if she has given birth and if so, at what age and how many. Hormone levels are intimately connected to stress levels, nutrition and environmental toxins.

Dr. Jerilynn C. Prior, researcher and professor of endocrinology at the University of British Columbia in Vancouver, Canada believes that the distressing symptoms that women experience in the time leading up to menopause are in fact due to the presence of estrogen dominance in her body. Her pioneering work revealed that an alarming number of women from their mid-thirties onward are anovulatory. The significance of her findings is vital in order to understand the real cause of the many distressing symptoms plaguing women as well as the most effective ways to address the problem.

Dr. Lee's clinical observations, reinforce Dr. Prior's findings. "Anovulatory cycles occur when for whatever reason, a women does not ovulate, therefore, does not produce a corpus luteum from which progesterone is made. Progesterone levels then drop dramatically allowing estrogen to dominate the hormonal environment. Although she is usually still menstruating, an anovulatory woman may have irregular cycles or changes in her menstrual flow. During the many months of anovulatory periods, estrogen production may become erratic with surges of inappropriately high levels, alternating with irregular low levels. These anovulatory cycles contribute to the many symptoms of estrogen dominance which include breast swelling and tenderness, mood swings, fatigue, little or no desire for sex, headaches, sleep disturbances, water retention and a tendency to put on weight. In addition, estrogen dominance interferes with the thyroid action which increases her fatigue, makes her feel cold all the time and contributes to her weight gain. The most common age for the initial stages of breast and uterine cancer is five years or more before menopause, well before estrogen levels fall but coinciding with a drop in progesterone."[4]

The stressful life-style that has become the norm in society takes a terrible toll on women's health. Stress is a major contributor to major hormonal imbalances. Chronic exhaustion is epidemic as women struggle to maintain a career, family and marriage. Quiet, nurturing time with herself is more a fantasy than a reality. In an effort to maintain her life-style, her adrenal glands are constantly pumping out hormones that were meant to be used sparingly or for "flight or fight" situations. All to often this leads them to become tired, sluggish and depleted. Dr. Lee comments on this condition. "Her body gets the message that survival is at stake., Blood sugar becomes unstable. Digestion goes awry so she isn't absorbing nutrients properly. The ovaries respond by shutting down in favor of survival. When her ovaries shut down, progesterone production occurs only at the adrenals but they aren't working and she's not getting any progesterone from poor dietary habits, so she becomes progesterone deficient and estrogen dominant."[5] Bingeing on sugar, caffeine and refined carbohydrates further exacerbates the problem leading to an impaired metabolism.

Toxic estrogens, known as xeno-estrogens or estrogen mimics, presently found in large quantities in the environment add to the estrogen excess. These sources include pesticides, herbicides, auto pollution, polychlorinated biphenyls (PCBs) and nonylphenols found in many detergents. Exposure to these chemicals may result in enlarged ovaries, possible ovarian tumors, breast cancer and premature "burnout" of ovarian follicles, contributing to an early menopause.

Males are not immune. Xeno-estrogens can contribute to atrophy of the testes, reduced sperm counts, small penises as well as cancer of the prostate and testes.

Anovulatory cycles also accelerate bone loss. Osteoporosis is the consequence of low progesterone levels since it is the bone building hormone. In combination with poor diet and lack of exercise, many women arrive at menopause with osteoporosis well under way, already having lost 25-30 percent of their bone mass.[6]

Unfortunately many peri-menopausal women are inappropriately diagnosed as having early menopause and thus prescribed HRT for their supposed "menopausal" symptoms. Taking more estrogen in addition to an already excess estrogen condition can not only lead to a worsening of the symptoms but can also contribute to more serious health problems. While hormonal problems are indeed widespread and a cause for concern, they are all too often symptoms of imbalance and poor health. Through reducing stress, improving diet and other life-style factors, using natural progesterone and receiving guidance from qualified practitioners of complimentary medicine, the peri-menopausal woman can quite naturally, safely and effectively alleviate and even eliminate her symptoms.

Symptoms which can be caused or made worse by Estrogen Dominance

Allergies

Altered thyroid activity (mimicking hypothyroidism

Auto immune disorders such as lupus and thyroiditis

Decreased sex drive

Depression

Dry Skin
Endometriosis
Excessive blood clotting
Fatigue
Fluid retention
Foggy thinking
Headaches
Heavy or irregular menses
Hirsutism (excessive hair growth on the body)
Impaired blood sugar control (hypoglycemia)
Increased body fat (especially around abdomen, hips and thighs)
Increased likelihood of fibrocystic breast disease and breast tenderness
Increased risk of endometrial cancer
Infertility
Loss of zinc and retention of copper
Memory loss
Miscarriage
Osteoporosis
PMS
Premenopausal bone loss
Reduced oxygen levels in all cells
Reduced vascular tone
Restraint of osteoclast function (ability to prevent the breakdown of bone tissue)
Thickened bile and gall bladder disease

Uterine fibroids

Uterine cramping

Effects of Estrogen Dominance*

1. When estrogen is not balanced by progesterone, it can pro-
    duce weight gain, headaches, bad temper, chronic fatigue
    and loss of interest in sex—all of which are part of the clini-
    cally recognized premenstrual syndrome.

2. Not only has it been well established that estrogen domi-
    nance encourages the development of breast cancer (thanks
    to estrogen's proliferative actions), it also stimulates breast
    tissue and can, in time, trigger fibrocystic breast disease—
    a condition which wanes when natural progesterone is
    introduced to balance the estrogen.

3. By definition, excess estrogen implies a progesterone de-
    ficiency. This, in turn, leads to a decrease in the rate of
    new bone formation in a woman's body by osteoblasts—
    the cells responsible for doing this job. Although most
    doctors are not yet aware of it, this is the prime cause of
    osteoporosis.

4. Estrogen dominance increases the risk of fibroids. One of
    the interesting facts about fibroids— often remarked on
    by doctors—is that regardless of size, fibroids commonly
    atrophy once menopause arrives and a woman's ovaries
    are no longer making estrogen. Doctors who commonly
    use progesterone with their patients have discovered that

giving a woman natural progesterone will also cause fibroids to atrophy.

5. In estrogen-dominant menstruating women where progesterone is not rising and falling in a normal way each month, the shedding of the womb lining doesn't take place. Menstruation becomes irregular. This condition can usually be corrected by making life-style changes and using a natural progesterone product. Estrogen dominance is easily diagnosed by having a doctor measure the level of progesterone through taking a saliva test.

6. Endometrial cancer (cancer of the womb) develops only where there is estrogen dominance or unopposed estrogen. This too can be prevented by the use of natural progesterone.

7. Waterlogging of the cells and an increase in intercellular sodium, which predisposes a woman to high blood pressure or hypertension, frequently occurs with estrogen dominance. This can also be a side effect of taking a synthetic progesterone. A natural progesterone cream usually clears up the problem.

8. The risk of stroke and heart disease is increased dramatically when a woman is estrogen dominant.

* Excerpt from *Passage to Power* by Leslie Kenton

Chapter 6

Adding Still Another Ingredient to the Hormone Soup

In addition to synthetic estrogens, women are now readily prescribed synthetic progestins, most commonly in the form of Provera. These progestins have been added to the estrogen formula to offset the hazards of estrogen drugs as previously mentioned. The pharmaceutical manufacturers themselves give a combined total of more than 120 potential risks and problems associated with HRT.[1]

At this point, it is important to make the distinction between the natural progesterone produced by the body and the synthetic progesterone-analogues classified as progestins, such as Provera, Duphaston, Primulut, Depo-Provera and Norplant. As you will learn, the two act differently in the body although doctors most often use the names 'progesterone' and 'progestin' interchangeably. Since natural progesterone is not a patentable product, the pharmaceutical companies have molecularly altered it to produce the synthetic progestins commonly used in contraceptives and HRT.

Synthetic progestins, because they are not exact replicas of the body's natural progesterone, unfortunately create a long list of side-effects, some of which can be quite severe. A partial list includes headaches, depression, fluid retention, increased risk of birth defects and early abortion, liver dysfunction, breast tenderness, breakthrough bleeding, acne, hirsutism (abnormal hair growth), insomnia, edema, weight changes, pulmonary embolism and premenstrual-like syndrome. Most importantly, progestins lack the intrinsic physiological benefits of progesterone and cannot function in the major biosynthetic pathways as progesterone does. Progestins actually disrupt many fundamental processes in the body. Progesterone is an essential hormone that also plays a part in the development of healthy nerve cells, brain function and thyroid function. Progestins tend to block the body's ability to produce and utilize natural progesterone to maintain these life-promoting functions.

To appreciate the scope of the side-effects of progestins, it is instructive to review the entry for medroxyprogesterone acetate (Provera) in the Physicians' Desk Reference (PDR). An abbreviated list from the 1995 PDR follows:

**Potential Side Effects of
Medroxyprogesterone Acetate (Provera)**

Warnings:

* Increased risk of birth defects such as heart and limb defects if taken during the first four months of pregnancy.
* Beagle dogs given this drug developed malignant mammary nodules.
* Discontinue this drug if there is sudden or partial loss of vision.
* This drug passes into breast milk, consequences unknown.
* May contribute to thrombophlebitis, pulmonary embolism and cerebral thrombosis.

Contraindications:

* Thrombophlebitis, thromboembolic disorders, cerebral apoplexy, liver dysfunction or disease, known or suspected malignancy of breast or genital organs, undiagnosed vaginal bleeding, missed abortion or known sensitivity.

Precautions:

* May cause fluid retention, epilepsy, migraine, asthma, cardiac or renal dysfunction.
* May cause breakthrough bleeding or menstrual irregularities.
* May contribute to depression.
* The effect of prolonged use of this drug on pituitary, ovarian, adrenal, hepatic and uterine function is unknown.
* May increase glucose tolerance; diabetic patients must be carefully monitored.
* May increase the thrombotic disorders associated with estrogen.

Adverse Reactions:

* May cause breast tenderness and galactorrhoea.
* May cause sensitivity reactions such as urticaria, pruritus, edema or rash.
* May cause acne, alopecia and hirsutism.
* Cervical erosions and changes in cervical secretions.
* Cholastic jaundice.

*   Mental depression, pyrexia, nausea, insomnia or somnolence.
*   Anaphylactic reactions and anaphylaxis (severe acute allergic reactions).
*   Thrombophlebitis and pulmonary embolism.
*   Breakthrough bleeding, spotting, amenorrhea or changes in menses.

When taken with estrogens, the following has been observed:

*   Rise in blood pressure, headache, dizziness, nervousness, fatigue.
*   Changes in sex drive, hirsutism and loss of scalp hair, decrease in T3 values (thyroid).
*   Premenstrual-like syndrome, changes in appetite.
*   Cystitis-like syndrome (urinary tact infections).
*   Erythema multiform, erythema nodosum, haemorrhagic eruption, itching.

In an article entitled, 'Risks of Estrogen and Progestins' in the December 1990 issue of *Maturitas*, an English-language medical journal, several serious side-effects were mentioned. The author, Dr. Marc L'Hermite, found that 5 to 7 percent of women on conjugated equine estrogen (Premarin) could develop severe high blood pressure. When HRT was withdrawn, the women would return to normal readings.

An even more chilling study was reported in the May, 1996 *American Health Consultant Fax Bulletin*. A recent study involving rhesus monkeys indicated that contraceptives containing progestins (Depo-Provera and Norplant) could cause vaginal changes which may increase the risk of HIV infection in women. Fourteen of eighteen rhesus monkeys who had progestin implants caught simian immune deficiency (a close cousin to HIV) after the virus was administered into the vagina of the monkeys. The researchers stress that, while an animal model can provide useful information, the result is not immediately transferable to humans. However, U.S. Public health officials must not be telling the whole truth since they are now encouraging all women on contraceptives to use condoms as well! What is most interesting about this study is the obvious conclusion that due to the implants of progestins, the monkeys' immune systems were seriously compromised, thus making them susceptible to the virus. Since monkeys do not go through menopause they are never depleted of progesterone— except when their normal progesterone-building capacity and progesterone receptors are blocked—as occurred in this study. In the same way that synthetic progesterone impaired the normal hormonal functioning of the monkeys, synthetic progesterone as found in the form of human birth control blocks the body's production of its natural progesterone. Immune system impairment can be one of the disturbing side-effects.

While it is argued that estrogen has beneficial cardiovascular effects by increasing the good HDL cholesterol, when progestin is added this effect is reversed. Harmful lipoprotein changes resulting from progestins have been enough in some studies to actually increase heart disease risk.[2]

The *Boston Nurses Questionnaire Study* showed in its latest findings that adding progestin to estrogen not only failed to reduce women's incidence of breast cancer, but actually increased it. The study showed that 10 years of use of estrogen alone increased the risk of breast cancer by 30-40 percent while women who took estrogen and progestin increased their risk of breast cancer by up to 100 percent.[3]

According to Dr. Neil Lauersen, in his book, *"PMS, Pre-menstrual Syndrome and You,"* one of the problems with synthetic progestins is that they inhibit a woman's concentration of natural progesterone in the blood and, in fact, worsen the imbalance of female hormones and intensify the symptoms of PMS. Some progestins are actually 2,000 times more potent than progesterone, which is why certain progestins can make women feel more out of sorts."

Chapter 7

And The Synthetic Hormones Just Keep Coming

The medical profession's and pharmaceutical industry's love affair with women's hormones now adds another 'wonder' hormone to the growing list. The latest new recruit is testosterone—in the synthetic and most unnatural variety known as methyl-testosterone. It is either administered on its own or in conjunction with estrogen.

While women do manufacture testosterone in their bodies—from natural progesterone—it is only found in very small amounts. In come cases, such as hysterectomies or extreme hormonal depletion, a low dose natural testosterone may have a limited role. However, it is not without negative effects.

Dr. Lee makes the point that the fact that testosterone is now being included in hormone treatment, particularly for increasing bone density, as protection from cardio-vascular disease and for treating fatigue, is an admission that estrogen by itself is not doing the job.

As is the case with all synthetic hormones, the side-effects of methyl-testosterone are quite alarming. Most of all, methyl-testosterone, which is administered either by injection or as a patch, is highly toxic to the liver, thus potentially causing serious liver damage or liver tumors. In addition, it can cause male pattern baldness, acne, excessive facial hair, enlarged clitoris and a permanent drop in voice pitch. There have been no conclusive studies showing the long-term safety of testosterone treatments.

Chapter 8

Hormone Addiction

Something which is little known about taking HRT is that it can be addictive. A former president of the London Royal College of Psychiatrists warns that estrogen used in HRT to counteract symptoms of menopause could be as addictive as heroin.[1]

In the 1970's testing was conducted on two groups of menopausal women. One group received estrogen replacement, the other group sugar pills (placebos). All were monitored for insomnia, nervousness, depression, dizziness, weakness, joint pain, palpitations, prickling sensations and hot flashes.

Both groups of women experienced an overall dramatic improvement during the first 90 days of the study, however the sugar pill group experienced more discomfort from hot flashes. When the groups were switched, those that had initially received estrogen experienced a pronounced return to their symptoms. It became apparent that once estrogen replacement stopped, a 'cold turkey' withdrawal effect was often experienced.

The same withdrawal effect has been found with implants, since the blood estradiol levels may become much higher than the body would normally produce.[2]

Nancy Beckham, herbalist, naturopath, homeopath and author of *Menopause: A Positive Approach Using Natural Therapies*, warns that, "Women on hormone replacement therapy who have enhanced well-being when their estradiol levels are very high but feel unwell when their blood levels are normal may be experiencing reactions similar to those of people on social drugs.

"It is well researched knowledge when you first have these drugs they give you a lift, which is pleasant; as you get used to the substance you find you need more to give you the same effect and ultimately your body craves a high level even though you may be unwell. When the substance in your blood drops below a certain level, you can experience withdrawal symptoms such as flashing, perspiration, sleep disturbance, shaking and other nervous reactions."[2]

While it is easy to prescribe HRT for women, there is hardly any medical data concerning the effects of stopping HRT in women who have received long-term treatment.[3] In one trial lasting three and a half years withdrawal lasted for six months.

Women must be advised to always taper off on their estrogen use and to never abruptly stop.

So, unbeknown to women, "menopause's little helper" could in fact be making estrogen junkies of them. It's great news for the pharmaceutical companies, but a calamity of untold proportion for women. Not only can they experience a wide range of physical symptoms, women may also suffer from psychiatric disturbances. Dr. Ellen Grant, author of *Sexual Chemistry*, was an early researcher of synthetic hormones and their effects on health. Dr. Grant has said, "when higher than expected rates of attempted suicide and violent deaths were recorded among HRT takers, the excuse was that more women suffering from depression are put on estrogens in attempt to treat them". Estrogens are rarely considered and therefore, overlooked as an extremely significant contributing factor in depressive behavior.

Chapter 9

Estrogen Dominance in the Environment

Another major factor contributing to an imbalance between estrogen and progesterone is environmental in nature. We, in the industrialized world, now live immersed in a rising sea of petrochemical derivatives. Petrochemicals are everywhere. They are in our air, food and water. Our machines run on petrochemicals, millions of products including plastics, microchips, medicines, clothing, foods, soaps, pesticides and even perfumes, are either made from petrochemicals or contain them. The popular slogan in the early 1950's, 'Better Living Through Chemistry', is returning to haunt us.

These organochlorine chemicals include pesticides, herbicides (such as DDT, DDE, dieldrin, atrazine, methoxychlor, hetachlor, kepone etc.) as well as various plastics (polycarbonated plastics found in baby bottles and water jugs). These chemicals have an uncanny ability to mimic natural estrogen. As estrogen mimics, these compounds are highly fat soluble, non-biodegradable, accumulate in fat tissue of animals and humans and are difficult to excrete. They are given the name xeno-estrogens since, although they are foreign chemicals, they are taken up by the estrogen receptor sites in the body, seriously interfering with natural biochemical changes.

Mounting research is now revealing an alarming situation world wide created by the inundation of these hormone mimics. A recently released book, *Our Stolen Future*, written by

Theo Colburn of the World Wild Life Fund, Dianne Dumanoski of the Boston Globe and John Peterson Meyers, a zoologist, have identified 51 hormone mimics, each able to unleash a torrent of effects such as reduced sperm production, cell division and sculpting the developing brain.[1] Acting as endocrine disrupters, these chemicals interfere with hormones to upset growth, development, behaviors, intelligence and reproductive capabilities.

Disturbing Changes

Extremely disturbing events are being reported globally about other alarming changes happening in the environment.

In 1947, orthnithologists noticed that eagles in Florida had lost their drive to mate and nest. In the 1960's ranch minks that were fed fish from Lake Michigan failed to reproduce. In 1977, female gulls in California were nesting with females.

Not long ago, in Lake Apopka in Florida, wildlife biologists discovered that strange biological occurrences were happening to the alligators living there. In 1980, a toxic spill occurred dumping huge amounts of a pesticide similar to DDT into the lake. That event was almost forgotten until five years later, when it was discovered that 90 percent of the alligators had disappeared. Most of those that remained were incapable of reproducing or had no urge to mate. The males were born with deformed penises that were 75 percent shorter than average. Further testing indicated that their testosterone levels were so low that they hormonally resembled females. Moreover, the females had abnormal ovaries and follicles described as "burned out".[2]

To add to this concern, recent reports show that strange hermaphroditic fish have been caught in Port Phillip Bay in Victoria, Australia. Similarly, a major British study revealed that male fish downstream from sewage treatment plants are changing sex as a result of estrogen chemicals which are not removed from treated effluent.[3]

Dr. Ana Soto, an endocrinologist at Tufts University, had been experimenting with cancer cells taken from human breasts and then cultured. She found that they would grow when they were fed estrogens. As part of her experiment she quit feeding the cells estrogen. To her total amazement, however, the cancer cells continued to grow for four months even when no estrogens were fed to them. Dr. Soto then realized that the manufacturer of the flasks she had been using had started to use a different plastic—one that, when it becomes warm, releases minute quantities of the estrogen-like compound nonylphenol! Nonylphenols refer to a family of compounds that are used as surfactants (reducing the surface tension of water creating a bridge between two chemicals that don't normally mix) in pesticides as well as industrial and institutional cleaning products. Her tissues samples were being contaminated by the xeno-estrogens of the plastic flasks![4]

The Israeli Breast Cancer Finding

The first well-publicized study was conducted by two scientist, Jerome Westin and Elihu Richter at the Hebrew University School of Medicine. They were interested in the what they called the "Israeli breast cancer anomaly". During the late 1970's and early 1980's, Israel's breast cancer rate, particularly in young women, was much higher than that of other countries. They were perplexed by these alarming statistics.

The study showed that three organochlorine pesticides that produced over a dozen types of cancers in ten different strains of rats and mice were present in extraordinarily high concentrations in Israeli milk and dairy products. The three - benzene hexachloride, lindane and DDT - were present for 10 years in concentrations up to 100 times greater than in American diary products at the time. Concentrations in Israeli breast milk were possibly 800 times greater than in American breast milk. Embryos, fetuses and infants were particularly vulnerable to the carcinogens. One report indicated that organochlorine pesticides accumulated in the fetus to levels more than 100 percent higher than those found in the mother.

After a tremendous public outcry, the government was forced to ban the three organochlorines. The result was a precipitous drop in concentrations of these substances in cow's milk and breast milk of up to 98 percent .

Breast cancer rates also went down dramatically. Of 28 European and Middle Eastern countries surveyed, only Israel recorded a true decrease in rates between 1976 and 1986. Westin and Richter believed that the drop in breast cancer resulted from this decline.

Another observation was made from this study: all known factors contributing to breast cancer affect estrogen. The connection is stated by Greenpeace, "Exposure to hormonally active organochlorines early in life, especially in utero when hormonal feedback systems are being imprinted, can result in permanent alteration of systems that control estrogen and other sex hormones. Studies show increased risk of breast cancer among women born to mothers with indications of high estrogen levels during pregnancy. Thus the transfer of accumulated organochlorines from mother to daughter may indeed contribute to breast cancer."[5]

The evidence is becoming indisputable. The legacy of this xeno-estrogenic pollution is permeating our very genes. There is an epidemic of reproductive abnormalities, including the steadily increasing number of breast, prostate, testicular and reproductive tract cancers, infertility, low sperm counts, poor sperm quality, the feminization of males and neurological disorders. The potential consequences of this over-exposure are staggering, especially considering that one of the consequences is passing on reproductive abnormalities to offspring.[5]

What the Future Portends

Just how serious is this problem? In a May 1993 article in the British Medical Journal, *Lancet*, researchers in Scotland and Denmark hypothesized that xeno-estrogens are responsible for a steadily declining sperm count in men. According to Neils Skakkebeak of the University of Copenhagen, sperm counts have dropped by more than 50 percent since 1940. Meanwhile, the rate of testicular and prostate cancer in the United States and Europe has tripled in the past 50 years. Reproductive abnormalities such as undescended testicles have become increasingly common. Xeno-estrogens have also been implicated in impaired brain development in children.[6] They are also directly implicated in the 30 to 80 percent increase in breast, ovarian and uterine cancers in women over the past fifty years.[7]

In some rural communities in Australia, where heavy pesticide use has left residuals in drinking water, there have been reports of boys with abnormally small penises, along with the feminization of males and the masculinization of females.

A German study has shown that women with endometriosis have significantly higher levels of chemicals known as PCB's in their bodies. Seventy years ago, only 21 cases of endometriosis had been reported in the world. Now there are over 5 million cases in the US alone. Another group of xeno-estrogens called nonylphenols appear in spermicides, in diaphragm jellies, on condoms and in vaginal gels to facilitate dispersal. This directly exposes the vagina and cervix to potent carcinogenic toxins.

A recent US Environment Protection Agency (EPA) data document revealed that US pesticide use reached an all-time high of 1,247 million pounds in 1995. This is over twice as much as was used 30 years ago when Rachel Carson's *Silent Spring* was published.[8] A study in the June 1996 edition of *Science* magazine showed that some combinations of hormone-distributing chemicals are much more powerful than any of the individual chemicals on their own. It revealed that combinations of two or three common pesticides, each at low levels which might be found in the environment, are up to 1,600 times as powerful together as any one individual pesticide by itself.

It is time for us to wake up and pay heed to these warnings for the sake of future generations. You can play your part in protecting your grandchildren and great-grand children in the same ways you can protect yourself: by refusing to use pesticides; minimizing your use of plastics, purchasing hormone-free meat and organic produce, using "green" products for detergents and household cleaners and in general using 'natural' products in favor of petrochemical products.

Recommended Reading:

Our Stolen Future, Theo Colburn, Dianne Dumanoski, John Peterson Myers, Dutton Publishers

The Feminization of Nature, Deborah Cadbury, Hamish Hamilton, London

Chapter　　　**10**

The Myth of Estrogen Deficiency

The trend these days is to strongly recommend hormone replacement therapy, featuring synthetic estrogens and progestins, to all menopausal women. Unfortunately, this enthusiasm for drugs is not backed up by the facts. Estrogen deficiency is loudly proclaimed by medical practitioners, pharmaceutical advertising and many lay publications as the primary cause of all the symptoms attributed to menopause and post menopause—mood swings, depression, hot flashes, vaginal dryness, loss of sex drive and accelerating osteoporosis.

But is there really such a thing as estrogen deficiency? While it is true that menopause is associated with decreasing estrogen levels, it is not known whether these decreased levels of estrogen do in fact cause all the symptoms of menopause. Dr. Carolyn DeMarco, author of *Take Charge of Your Body* and a physician specializing in women's health issues, states, "there is no direct proof that estrogen lack causes heart disease or other ailments associated with the menopause".

Germaine Greer, writes that, "the proponents of HRT have never proved that there is an estrogen deficiency nor have they explained the mechanism by which the therapy of choice effected its miracles. They have taken the improper course of defining a disease from its therapy."

Dr. Jerilynn C. Prior points out that no study proving the

relationship between estrogen deficiency and menopausal symptoms and related diseases has yet been done. "Instead," says Dr. Prior, "a notion has been put forward that since estrogen levels go down, this is the most important change and explains all the things that may or may not be related to menopause. So estrogen treatment at this stage of our understanding is premature. This is a kind of backwards science. It leads to ridiculous ideas—like calling a headache an aspirin deficiency disease."[1]

Considering that western women tend to have a 10-15 year period prior to menopause when they are estrogen dominant and suffering from estrogen dominance symptoms, why are their doctors prescribing them still more estrogen?

During menopause, estrogen levels decrease to one-half to one-third of pre-menopausal baseline levels. While estrogen production falls only 40 - 60 percent, progesterone levels on the other hand, fall close to zero when ovulation no longer occurs.[2] Would it not be wiser to consider the progesterone loss effect when evaluating post menopausal symptoms and related conditions such as osteoporosis, heart disease, depression and loss of sex drive?

According to David Zava, PhD, director of research at Aeron Life Cycle Laboratory, who is developing saliva testing methods for monitoring levels of phytohormones in food and in the body, "It is interesting to note that Asian women have so few menopausal symptoms, despite the fact that their estrogen levels are, on average, only half the levels of Western women. Epidemiological studies suggest that diets high in soy foods, common in Asian countries are associated with less cancer, heart disease and osteoporosis.

"Hot flashes are not common in Asian countries. Pre and post menopausal Asian women have only about half the circulating levels of estradiol and estrone (high levels are associated with an increased risk of breast cancer risk) in their bodies compared to American women. This might be the reason why they have a three to five-fold lower incidence of breast cancer.

"A recent paper by Lee-Jane Lu confirms that it is phytoestrogens in soy that are responsible for lowering estradiol levels. Soy phytoestrogens serve as a surrogate estrogen in their bodies and we think this is the reason they don't have cancer and they don't have heart disease and significant osteoporosis. Asian women don't get endometrial cancer and men don't get prostate cancer."

The 'estrogen deficiency' hypothesis, as an explanation of most menopausal symptoms or health problems, is thus not supported by the facts of estrogen blood levels, by world wide ecological studies or by endocrinology experts. Has everyone jumped onto the 'estrogen deficiency' bandwagon without really understanding what is happening to women's hormones?

Chapter 11

But My Blood Tests Say...

Part of the confusion around HRT lies in the accepted way of measuring estrogen. Every woman who finds herself at the doctor's office suffering from menopausal symptoms will be given a blood serum test to determine her hormone levels. Serum is the clear, watery part of the blood without any of the red blood cells. When the ovaries make estrogen and progesterone for circulation in the watery blood serum, they bind them to protein to make them more water soluble. Protein-bound hormones are not biologically active, however they represent over 90 percent of the hormones found in blood serum.[1]

What does all this mean? It means that, for the most part, blood tests to accurately measure the levels of hormones in a woman's body are useless and extremely unreliable. It is likely that your doctor may be unaware of this. The tests are only able to measure 1-9 percent of the biologically active hormones circulating in the body. Ninety percent or more remains undetected by these tests! So most readings that may show low estrogen levels aren't measuring what's really there. Of course, the danger comes when a woman is prescribed hormones based upon test results which are erroneous. Even though her blood test may show low levels of estrogen, from which her doctor concludes she needs more estrogen (resulting in a prescription for estrogen), it is often the last thing in the world her body really needs.

"One prominent Californian gynecologist, skilled in prescribing hormones, finally stopped trying to measure blood levels and began relying on a woman's description of the way she was feeling. She found this to be more accurate because blood levels varied so widely during a woman's cycle."[2]

Dr. Susan Love concurs. She says, "Blood tests for hormones are notoriously unreliable. Although (saliva testing) is a good way to measure them, I don't know why you would want to. There is no optimal estrogen level - only one which feels right for you. The dose of hormones you take should be balanced against your symptoms and not some arbitrary laboratory number determined by blood or saliva."[3]

So, how do you accurately test hormone levels? It is called 'saliva testing'. Hormones present in saliva reflect only the biologically available hormones. Saliva hormone tests are less expensive, very accurate and more relevant than serum tests for checking the accurate levels of hormones. It is able to confirm that any hormones being taken are being absorbed and utilized. Five years ago the World Health Organization began using saliva testing in place of blood serum testing.

If your doctor is unable to provide you with a saliva test, they can be ordered directly from the laboratories. You will then need to send your saliva test to the testing lab. The lab will check your saliva for hormone levels and send the results back to you. It is recommended that you discuss the confirmed results with your doctor.

Saliva tests and kits for both hormone and bone assays can be ordered from:

Aeron Life Cycle Laboratory
1933 Davis Street - Suite 310
San Leandro, California 94577
Phone: (510) 729-0375   Fax: (510) 729 0383

Great Smokies Diagnostic Laboratory
18a Regent Park Boulevard
Asheville, North Carolina 28806
Phone: 704-253-0621
Fax: 704-253-1127
E-mail: cs@gsdl.com

Chapter 12

The Pill—A Bitter Pill To Swallow

With hindsight, it will very likely be recorded in history that the widespread prescribing of synthetic hormones to women was the biggest medical bungle of the century. Most women taking oral contraceptives have very little idea about the hormones they are putting into their bodies, nor are they knowledgeable about the potentially serious side-effects.

A revolution was about to begin when the birth control pill arrived on the scene in 1960. It heralded an era that would emancipate fertile women from the burden of unwanted pregnancies thus opening the door to greater equality and freedom. For the past 40 years about 200 million women around the world have chosen the Pill as their preferred method of contraception. This "medical miracle" has enlisted almost 90 per cent of western women of reproductive age on some kind of contraceptive at some time in their lives.

The choices of the steroid hormone contraceptive has now expanded to include the combined and the low dose pill made with estrogen and synthetic progesterone called progestin or the mini pill either in the form of an implant or injection made only with progestins such as Depo-Provera or Norplant.

The Pill has been proclaimed as one of the most studied drugs in history. After three decades of experimentation (unfortunately on the unsuspecting pill users), we are told safe dosages are, at last, finally known. However, as the thin veneer of advertising hype, pharmaceutical cover-ups and sanitized clinical trials is peeled away, another picture emerges revealing the devastating consequences to women's health and well-being from the use of steroid hormones found in the Pill

So, just what are the effects of suppressing natural hormones with synthetic ones? The Pill literally stops menstruation and bleeding only occurs each month because the synthetic hormones are not taken for seven days of the cycle. The bleeding that occurs would be more accurately termed 'withdrawal bleeding' not menstruation.

Taking the combined Pill increases the risk of coronary artery disease, breast cancer, cervical cancer, infertility, strokes, nutritional deficiencies and high blood pressure. The side-effects include nausea, vomiting, migraine-type headaches, breast tenderness, weight increases, changes in sex drive, depression, head hair loss, facial hair growth blood clots and increased incidence of vaginitis. Also, women with a history of epilepsy, migraine, asthma or heart disease may find that their symptoms worsen. Many of these effects may persist long after the discontinuation of the Pill.

According to Nancy Beckham, in her book *Menopause—A Positive Approach to Natural Therapies*, "Women on the Pill have a greater tendency to liver dysfunction and to more allergies. Estrogen drugs also affect vitamin concentrations. Vitamin A levels may be raised in the blood; vitamin B12 and C may be lowered. The clinical significance is not yet known." In addition essential fatty acids and zinc are depleted.

The introduction of Depo-Provera and Norplant, both of which are made from synthetic progestins, are equally disturbing to a woman's hormonal health, with all the previously listed side-effects and risks of progestins.

It is common practice today and has been for over a generation to prescribe birth control pills to women who complain of menstrual-related irregularities or discomfort. Under the prevailing misunderstanding about the real cause of women's problems, it is no wonder that this is the most accepted form of treatment. But, it's not really a treatment at all. It does not address the underlying imbalance—physiological and often emotional—which relates to estrogen dominance, poor diet and emotional stress.

It is important to recognize that the Pill is a potent artificial steroid drug which carries serious risks to a woman's health. Teenagers are especially vulnerable. The Pill is broken down in the liver which is consequently exposed to high doses of steroids. According to a report in the November 1995 *Natural Fertility Management* newsletter, the Pill causes 150 chemical changes in a girl's body. Many of these are not fully understood. The Pill seriously compromises a teenager's health, predisposing her to a lifetime of health problems. Teenager's need to be very fit and healthy to withstand all the metabolic changes in their bodies caused by the Pill.

The prevailing myth that the Pill is a safe and natural way to correct hormonal imbalances has lead to its widespread use in correcting teenager's menstrual cycles or alleviating painful periods. Puberty has now been medicalized. Even though nature often requires several years to help balance out a teenager's menstrual cycle, girls, as young as eleven years old, complaining of irregularities will all too often be recommended the Pill to supposedly help "regulate" their periods. Such common practices are both irresponsible and highly dangerous.

Since the breast tissue of young girls is still developing and is particularly sensitive to the over-stimulation from synthetic estrogen, the earlier a woman uses the Pill the greater the risk not only of developing breast cancer but also large tumors and a worse prognosis.

In a study by Olsson (*Cancer 1991)* it was shown that the Pill caused chromosomal aberrations in the breast tissue of young female users.

One study found the most terrifying results: the younger the women were at the time of diagnosis, the greater the possibility they would be dead within five years. John Wilks, author of *"A Consumer's Guide to the Pill and Other Drugs"* sums up this scandalous abuse of steroid hormones by stating that, "Given these results, it is not beyond the bounds of reasoned argument to suggest that this situation could be categorized as drug- induced vandalism of the female physiology. Yet little or nothing is heard of this lamentable betrayal of young women's health."[2]

Instead of relying upon the Pill to "regulate" problem periods, girls would be much better off to correct the problem at its source through improved diet, nutritional supplements, exercise and attending to emotional stresses. It would save them from the horrors of breast cancer and the high risk of dying from the disease.

A word is needed here about the trend that is occurring in our culture of early puberty in girls. According to Dr. Lee, "Early puberty results in longer lifetime exposure to estrogen produced by the ovaries, thus increasing cancer risk. It also appears that it leads to earlier follicle burnout and anovulatory cycles (menstruation without ovulation), starting as early as the mid thirties for most women. Just a generation or two ago, teenage girls didn't reach puberty until their late teens. Now they may start menstruating as early as 11 or 12. We have come to think of this as normal. It's not!

My suspicion is that this early onset of puberty is caused by exposure to the estrogens and xeno-estrogens so prevalent in every part of our environment from our meat supply (hormones are used throughout the meat industry in nearly all Western industrialized countries) to the air we breathe."

Francesca Naish, author of the book, *Natural Fertility*, reports that a 10-year program by the California Walnut Creek drug study of hospital admissions reports significantly increased inflammatory diseases in women under 40 who have taken or currently take the Pill. These inflammatory conditions include respiratory, digestive, urogenital and musculoskeletal disorders.

She goes on to say that, "The residue of the Pill can take three to six months to be eliminated from the system. This is the minimum amount of time that should lapse between coming off the Pill and conceiving, otherwise there are increased risks of fetal deformities.

"The Mini-Pill, which contains only progestins, is also often prescribed for lactating mothers and has been shown to severely deplete the nutrients available for the child in the mother's milk as well as providing the baby with an overdose of synthetic hormones. Synthetic progesterone is known to act on the hypothalamus, an important brain center and may masculinize a female infant and contribute to neo-natal jaundice."

We are only just beginning to realize the price we are paying for being part of a culture where fast food, fast cures and fast sex predominate. Certainly the long term effects of the Pill, in whatever form it comes, is still to be fully determined, not to mention the effects it may have on future generations. Is it worth the price that women must pay in terms of their physical, emotional and mental health for this form of contraception?

Most women will ask, "Well, just what are the natural alternatives to the Pill?" Barrier methods such as the diaphragm, condom and spermicide are certainly effective options. However, the most profound answer to that question requires a woman to gain a deeper understanding of the workings of her body and her natural cycles. It's learning about the various indications of fertile and non-fertile times. Owning one's fertility means to have an intimate relationship with one's own body. It requires taking responsibility for sexual intercourse. It also requires the ability to communicate with an understanding and receptive partner. It certainly is a totally different approach from the way most women address the issue of contraception and for that matter sexual relationships. It may require more effort but the benefits are immense.

Perhaps it is time for women to rethink the entire Pill issue. Two important questions worth asking are: "How precious is your health?" and "Are you willing to learn safe, natural forms of contraception?" The change that is needed to stop the exploitation of women's health for profits will require women as well as conscientious health professionals to make new, informed and safe choices. The health and well-being of millions of women around the world and the health of future generations depends on it.

Side-Effects of the Pill

Minor (non-life threatening)

Allergic reactions
Breakthrough bleeding
Decreased immune system function
Disturbances in liver function
Eye disorders such as double vision, swelling of optic nerve,
    contact lens intolerance and corneal inflammation

Facial and body hair growth
Fluid retention and bloating
Fungal infections and tinea
Hair loss
Hayfever, asthma, skin rashes
Loss of libido
Lumpy or tender breasts
Migraines
Nausea
Psychological and emotional disorders, depression,
    mood changes
Secretions from the breast
Skin discoloration
Suicide is much more common among Pill-users than
    those using other forms of contraception
Weight gain
Systemic candida infection (candida or yeast infection)
Urinary tract infection
Venereal warts
Vaginal discharges, including a much greater
    tendency to have vaginal thrush
Varicose veins

Major Side-Effects

Disturbance to blood-sugar metabolism (possibly
    contributing to diabetes or hypoglycemia)
Greatly increased chance of suffering a stroke

(increasing with age and duration of Pill usage)
Increased chance of hardening of the arteries and
    high blood pressure
Increased risk of blood clots
Increased risk of gall bladder disease (gall stones)
Liver tumors (increasing with duration of Pill usage)
Possible link with cancer of the endometrium, cervix,
    ovaries, liver and lungs
Significantly increased risk of ectopic pregnancy
Strong probability of more rapid development of
    pre-existing cancers and progression to cancer of
    abnormal cells
Three-to-six fold increase in risk of heart attacks
    (according to age)
Osteoporosis

If you are presently on the Pill and wish to continue, it is
extremely important to understand that the synthetic progestin in it will be taken up by all the progesterone receptor sites.
Since progestins are synthetic analogues which means they
are not exact matches of natural progesterone, they may interfere with the many bodily functions regulated by natural
progesterone. It is no wonder that the Pill has such a long list
of side-effects. Therefore, according to Dr. Lee, natural progesterone will have only limited or, in some cases, no benefit since
the synthetic progestins have already and will continue to 'use
up' the progesterone receptor sites.

Recommended Reading:

1. *Natural Fertility*, Francisca Naish,
   Crossing Press, California

2. *A Cooperative Method of Birth Control*,
   Margaret Nofzeger,
   Book Publishing Company, (1 800 695-2241)

For further information about Natural Fertility
Management Training's and other products and services
 contact:

Natural Fertility Management
P. O. Box 2215
Chapel Hill, N.C. 27515
Internet email: stahmann@yahoo.com

Chapter 13

Enter Natural Progesterone

The present day prospects for a woman's health would indeed be gloomy if there were no other alternatives available. Fortunately, this is not the case. There exists a huge range of effective options. But to discover them, it is vital to look elsewhere than the traditional allopathic medical model. There is a long history of very successful treatments based upon a more natural approach to addressing the underlying symptoms. These include Naturopathy, Homeopathy, Traditional Chinese Medicine, Chiropractic, Herbalism and many more.

One of the most significant treatments presently available that safely and effectively addresses women's hormonal imbalances and related health problems is natural progesterone. In the early 1900's, research into the mysteries of women's hormones first revealed the existence of estrogen. Further investigations identified a second hormone which was proven to be necessary for a successful pregnancy, thus it was named progesterone (i.e. pro-gestation). Initial experiments extracted progesterone from sows' ovaries. It was then discovered that the placenta synthesized large amounts of progesterone. In the late 1930's, experimental work and clinical applications used progesterone obtained from the harvesting of placentas after childbirth and quick freezing them to extract the progesterone.

By 1939 it was discovered that an ingredient called

diosgenin in the Mexican wild yam (Dioscorea villosa)—not to be confused with the average supermarket yam which is really a sweet potato—could be converted very easily and inexpensively into a molecule which is identical to the progesterone the body makes, now known as natural progesterone.

PMS is Real

The research and writings in the 1950's by pioneering British gynecologist, Dr. Katherina Dalton, first identified and coined the phrase 'Premenstrual Syndrome' (PMS). She was also the first to widely use progesterone with her patients. Dr. Dalton came to use progesterone through personal experience. She had noticed that her menstrual migraines disappeared during the last six months of her pregnancy when progesterone levels naturally soar. She first experimented on herself, discovering her migraines disappeared, and then found rapid and unequivocal effects when used with her women patients.

Thus began her decades-long and very vocal advocacy of this now international treatment. Since 1953, Dr. Dalton has become a leading investigator into PMS and a respected authority in the field. Besides establishing PMS as the most common of women's endocrine disorders, she was the first to show that PMS is the result of a progesterone deficiency and can be eliminated by increasing the levels of natural progesterone.

Progesterone Remembered

One present crusader committed to dispelling the erroneous beliefs about the cause and treatment of hormonal imbalance is Dr. John Lee. After 30 years of practice, Dr. Lee found that the women he saw through their child bearing years were now going through menopause and experiencing osteoporosis.

In 1982, after studying the work of biochemist, Ray Peat, Ph.D., on the importance of natural progesterone in bodily functions, Dr. Lee began using a transdermal natural progesterone cream derived from the wild yam to treat his osteoporotic patients.

He claims that, "After I had been in practice about 20 years, I had more and more people who had osteoporosis. In 1976 and 1978, it became apparent to everybody in medicine that estrogen therapy, as we were instructed to give for osteoporosis, not only was not working very well for their bones, but was the only known cause of cancer of the uterus. "In my practice, I asked women who had osteoporosis to take the natural progesterone cream and I followed their bone mineral density tests just to see what would happen.

"It turned out that in three years time, the women typically gained 15 percent more bone. It wasn't just merely a delay of the osteoporosis, the bones actually became better. And in the process of following these women, I learned all the other things that progesterone did for them. They reported to me that fibrocystic breasts turned back to normal. Those that had acne or hair loss, male pattern baldness, showed me that their hair was coming back. These were things that at first I found unbelievable and yet when I researched them in our hospital library, to find references to see if anyone had studied them, I found that, yes, they had been studied and, yes, they were known effects of progesterone."[1]

Dr. Lee, further states that, along with increased bone density, these women were being relieved of their PMS, fibrocystic breast disease, hot flashes, vaginal dryness, depression, hypertension, migraines, hypothyroidism, high cholesterol and other menopausal symptoms.

Dr. Lee became even more convinced of the efficacy of natural progesterone when he found that many women could decrease their estrogen and finally discontinue it entirely and still maintain their bone density. Though estrogen is often deemed necessary for vaginal dryness and hot flashes, he also saw these problems improved with just the use of natural progesterone.

For the past fifteen years, Dr. Lee has conducted independent research into the many applications of natural progesterone. His non-pharmaceutically funded research presents a much broader understanding of a woman's hormonal options and offers a totally safe, effective alternative that is free of all side effects. Together with a good diet and some life-style changes, he has found that this natural hormone is capable of eliminating much of the suffering associated with both PMS and menopause.

A Recurring Theme

Dr. Lee's research led him to the realization that there was a consistent theme running through women's complaints of the distressing and often debilitating symptoms of PMS, perimenopause and menopause — the presence of too much estrogen in the body (estrogen dominance). He was convinced that, instead of estrogen playing its essential role within the well balanced symphony of steroid hormones, it overshadowed the other players, creating biochemical dissonance. Adding more estrogen to a woman's body, either in the form of contraceptives or HRT, was the last thing she needed.

However, the prevailing myth of estrogen deficiency means that when estrogen dominant symptoms appear, such as hot flashes, menstrual difficulties, depression etc., guess what is prescribed? More estrogen! The delicate natural estrogen/progesterone balance is radically altered due to too much estrogen. Progesterone deficiency is then exacerbated.

For many years, Dr. Lee has been sounding the alarm, with little support and much resistance from his medical colleagues.

However, while the erroneous focus has been on estrogen, natural progesterone seems to have been totally overlooked by medical science. Considering that natural progesterone is non-patentable and inexpensive, it is not surprising that this is so. It is important, however, to have a much greater understanding of and appreciation for this remarkable hormone.

It is also important to remember that it is progesterone that is responsible for maintaining the secretory endometrium which is necessary for the survival of the embryo as well as the developing fetus throughout gestation. It is little realized, however, that progesterone is the mother of all hormones. Progesterone is the important precursor in the biosynthesis of adrenal corticosteroids (hormones that protect against stress) and of all sex hormones (testosterone and estrogen). This means that progesterone has the capacity to be turned into other hormones further down the biochemical pathways as and when the body needs them. The point needs to be emphasized that estrogen and testosterone are end metabolic products made from progesterone. Without adequate progesterone, estrogen and testosterone will not be sufficiently available to the body. Besides being a precursor to sex hormones, progesterone also provides many other important intrinsic physiological functions.

Supplementation with natural progesterone corrects the real problem—progesterone deficiency. It is not known to have any side-effects nor have any toxic levels been found to date. Natural progesterone increases libido, protects against fibrocystic breast disease, helps protect against breast and uterine cancer, maintains the lining of the uterus, hydrates and oxygenates the skin, reverses facial hair growth and thinning of the hair, acts as a natural diuretic, helps to eliminate depression and increases a sense of well-being, encourages fat burning and the use of stored energy, normalizes blood clotting and is a precursor to other important stress and sex hormones. Even the two most prevalent menopausal symptoms, hot flashes and vaginal dryness, quickly disappear with applications of natural progesterone.

Thus progesterone has many diverse and beneficial actions throughout the body. Since progesterone protects against the undesirable side effects of unopposed estrogen, whether produced by the body before menopause or as a consequence of estrogen supplementation or xeno-estrogens from the environment, it will assist the body to return to greater hormonal balance. All of the undesirable effects of estrogen are countered by progesterone. Restoring proper progesterone levels is restoring hormonal balance.

Functions of Progesterone

*   is a precursor of the other sex hormones, including estrogen and testosterone.

* maintains secretory endometrium (uterine lining).
* is necessary for the survival of the embryo and fetus throughout gestation.
* protects against fibrocystic breast disease.
* is a natural diuretic.
* helps use fat for energy.
* functions as a natural antidepressant.
* helps thyroid hormone action.
* normalizes blood clotting.
* restores sex drive.
* helps normalize blood sugar levels.
* normalizes zinc and copper levels.
* restores proper cell oxygen levels.
* protects against endometrial cancer.
* helps protect against breast cancer.
* assists to builds bone and is protective against osteoporosis.
* is a precursor of cortisone synthesis (in the adrenal cortex).
* reverses hirsutism (excessive hair growth).

Chapter 14

Discovering Some of the
Benefits of Natural Progesterone

Clinical research and personal experience are presenting more and more convincing evidence about the multiple roles natural progesterone plays in the body. Many important discoveries about progesterone's place in creating and maintaining health have been forgotten along the way, overshadowed by estrogen's starring role.

One of the problems with medicine is that it tends to label hormones by their presumed functions, thus there is the tendency to classify hormones either as sex hormones or thyroid hormones, etc. However, the body is a more complex and interrelated organism—hormones do so many things. For instance, brain cells concentrate progesterone and testosterone to levels 20 times higher than the blood carries. Imagine, progesterone receptors in the brain! Obviously brain cells wouldn't do this unless progesterone and testosterone has some important job to do there. This latest research helps to unravel the curious findings from many of Dr. Lee's patients who reported increased concentration, mental alertness and other improved mental abilities while using progesterone! Perhaps the foggy thinking so often associated with menopause is merely another sign of progesterone deficiency.

Growing interest is stimulating the enthusiasm for more research. It might even be said that at long last progesterone is coming of age! Without a doubt, more information about progesterone's role in creating health will be revealed in the years ahead. The following are some of the known benefits natural progesterone provides.

Aches and Pains of the Muscles (Fibromyalgia)

When stretching any distance, nerve cells are sheathed in an off-white insulating covering called myelin which protects the nerves from trauma and chemical erosion as well as preventing short-circuiting of the electric impulses along the way. Along the nerves throughout the body are special cells called Schwann cells which continually maintain the myelin sheath. Progesterone is made by the Schwann cells, allowing them to perform their function.

It is no surprise, then, to discover that fibromyalgia, inflammation of the nerve cells in the muscle accompanied by aches and pains, is the result of a progesterone deficiency. The traditional medical approach uses non-steroid anti-inflammatory drugs, anti-depressants and a variety of stress management techniques without great success. Dr. Lee found that fibromyalgia, which is reaching epidemic proportions in the United States, would disappear within six months to a year upon using progesterone supplements.

Allergies

Allergies are produced in the body when the allergen (the allergy-producing substance) load exceeds the capacity of the body to deal with it. Adequate cortisone blocks the histamine response to allergens. Progesterone is a precursor not only to estrogen and testosterone, but also to all the corticosteroids made by the adrenal glands. Adrenal exhaustion is the result of stress, vitamin C deficiency and progesterone deficiency. Progesterone assists in alleviating allergy problems.

Arthritis

Arthritis is a condition of aching joints or an ache of the connective tissue around the joints. Doctors usually prescribe non-steroid anti-inflammatory drugs. The origins of such symptoms have a variety of causes. One such cause is the lack of physiological (made by the body) cortisone responses to check the inflammatory reactions. Natural progesterone has anti-inflammatory properties that the synthetic analogues do not have. In addition to his own experience, Dr. Lee, has had many doctors report that women have experienced significant relief from aches and pains.

Auto Immune Disorders

Auto immune disorders occur when one's own antibodies attack the organs and tissues in the body. Auto immune disorders are generally found more often in women. The onset of such disorders, such as Lupus, Graves' Disease, Hashimoto's thyroiditis or Sjirgren's disease are more prevalent in middle age and are related to estrogen supplementation or estrogen dominance. Recent studies have shown that women who use hormone replacement therapy are more likely to get lupus.[1]

Hormone researcher, Dr. Ray Peat, professor of biochemistry

at Blake College in Oregon has found, "The thymus gland is the main regulator of the immune system. Estrogen causes it to shrink while progesterone protects it."[2]

Candida

A common problem for many women these days is a condition called candida. It is the proliferation of yeast growth due to several factors. Vaginal cells contain glucose which is a favorite nutrient of candida. Estrogen dominance increases mucus glucose levels, encouraging candida growth. When hormonal imbalance is restored to normal balance using progesterone, candida growth is less likely to persist.

Endometriosis

A serious condition in which tiny islets of endometrium (the inner lining of the uterus) become scattered in areas where they don't belong—the fallopian tubes, within uterine musculature and on the outer surface of the uterus and other pelvic organs, the colon, the bladder and the sides of the pelvic cavity.

With each monthly cycle, these islets of endometrium respond to ovarian hormones exactly as endometrial cells do within the uterus—they increase in size, swell with blood and bleed into the surrounding tissue at menstruation. The bleeding (no matter how minor) into the surrounding tissue causes inflammation and is very painful. Symptoms begin 7 to 12 days before menstruation and become excruciatingly painful during menstruation.

Sometimes doctors will recommend the radical decision of a hysterectomy for severe cases of endometriosis. All other options should be fully explored first. A hysterectomy is a major trauma for a woman's body. Dr. Lee has had considerable success treating endometriosis with natural progesterone. "Since we know that estrogen initiates endometrial cell proliferation and the formation of blood vessel accumulation in the endometrium, the aim of the treatment is to block this monthly estrogen stimulus to the aberrant endometrial islets. Progesterone stops further proliferation of endometrial cells."

Dr. Lee advises women to use natural progesterone cream from day six of the cycle to day 26 each month, using one ounce of cream per week for three weeks, stopping just before their period begins. This treatment requires patience. Over time (four to six months), however, the monthly pain gradually subsides as monthly bleeding in these islets lessens and healing of the inflammation occurs.[3]

It is interesting to note that endometriosis is cured by menopause due to reduced estrogen levels.

As previously mentioned, there is also a connection between increased xeno-estrogens, particularly nonylphenols and endometriosis. Considering that endometriosis is a twentieth century disease, it is obvious that environmental factors should be seriously considered.

Christiane Northrup, M.D., author of *Women's Bodies, Women's Wisdom*, considers endometriosis an illness of competition. She believes that "it comes about when a woman's emotional needs are competing with her functioning in the outside world. When a woman feels that her innermost emotional needs are in direct conflict with what the world is demanding of her, endometriosis is one of the ways in which her body tries to draw her attention to the problem.

A great many of the women I've seen who have endometriosis drive themselves relentlessly in the outer world, rarely resting, rarely tuning in to their innermost needs and deepest desires."[4]

Fibroids

Fibroids are round, firm, benign (non-cancerous) lumps on the uterine wall, composed of smooth muscle and connective tissue. They are rarely found singularly. While they are usually small in size, they can grow to the size of a grapefruit. They often cause, or are coincidental with, heavier periods, irregular bleeding and/or painful periods. More than 40 percent of women over the age of fifty have these benign growths. They are also the most common reason for performing a hysterectomy and usually the most unwarranted reason.

Dr. Lee states that fibroid tumors are, " Another example of estrogen dominance secondary to anovulatory cycles and consequent progesterone deficiency. They generally occur 8 to 10 years before menopause."[5]

Natural progesterone offers a better alternative. Fibroids are a product of estrogen dominance, which is why they disappear after menopause. However, if estrogen is supplied after menopause, fibroid tumors will be stimulated to grow. When sufficient natural progesterone is replaced, fibroid tumors no longer grow in size and often will shrink. Natural progesterone used in conjunction with dietary changes which includes a high fibre, low fat, primarily vegetarian and organic diet is quite effective in reducing fibroids. Other natural remedies which include Western herbs, homeopathic remedies and Chinese herbs have also provided successful treatment.

Hair Loss and Increased Facial Hair

Through lack of ovulation (anovulatory cycles) progesterone levels fall. The decrease in progesterone signals the adrenals to increase the production of an androgen (male-like) hormone called androstenedione. This adrenal cortical steroid produces male characteristics such as male pattern hair loss and increased facial hairs especially the dark ones appearing on the chin. When progesterone levels are raised through the use of natural progesterone, the adrenal hormone production will gradually fall. Although it usually takes four to six months to restore normal hair growth patterns, head hair will grow and facial hair will disappear. Increased androstenedione levels at menopause contribute to the thinning of hair and increase facial hairs of postmenopausal women. Along with an improved diet and proper nutrition, natural progesterone cream will help reverse this condition.

High Blood Pressure

Estrogen dominance is one of the many causes of high blood pressure or hypertension. Estrogens and progestins adversely affect cell membranes. Milton Crane has extensively studied the effects of estrogen, progestins and progesterone on cell membranes and high blood pressure. He has concluded that estrogen dominance and oral contraceptives are a major cause of hypertension in women.[6]

If you are on diuretics or other anti-hypertensive drugs and using progesterone, it is wise to have your doctor monitor your blood pressure, so as to reduce or eliminate your anti -hypertensive drugs gradually as appropriate to prevent low blood pressure.

Estrogen dominance or synthetic progestins substituting for progesterone impair the functioning of cell membranes, causing increased levels of sodium and water in the cells. This results in intracellular edema, a build up of fluids in the cells leading to hypertension. Dr. Lee estimates that 90 percent of all cases of essential hypertension are probably due to unrecognized hormonal imbalance.

Hot Flashes

Hot flashes are one of the most prevalent symptoms of hormonal change in western culture. It is interesting to note that Japanese women do not experience hot flashes and, in fact, have no word for it. As menopause is approached and even 5 to 10 years afterwards, it is estimated that around 80 percent of western women experience this sudden rise of heat in the body, with up to 40 percent suffering sufficiently to seek assistance from a health professional.

The hot flash is still not totally understood. Diminished estrogen levels play a role. Withdrawal of estrogen causes an increase in the levels of the hormones FSH and LH. The brain center that regulates the secretion of these hormones, the hypothalamus, directs many body functions including body temperature, sleep patterns, metabolic rate, mood and reaction to stress. The higher the levels of FSH and LH, the more blood vessels dilate or enlarge, raising body temperature, which increases blood flow to the skin—the hot flash.

The part of the hypothalamus involved in these hormonal changes monitors progesterone as well as estrogen. Since the post menopausal woman continues to make estrogen in respectable levels and makes little or no progesterone, hot flashes may respond well to progesterone supplementation alone. Hot flashes will also respond to much smaller levels of supplemental estrogen when progesterone is added.

Not all hot flashes are related to decreases in estrogen levels. Hypothyroidism can be a cause, as can alcohol intake and out-of-control diabetes. In fact, waves of heat may hit anyone, of any age, who engages in behavior that forces the temperature-regulating system to step up its activities.

The most common triggers for hot flashes include spicy foods, caffeine, chocolate, alcohol, drugs of all kinds, hot drinks, hot weather and stress. Irregular eating can also destabilize your blood sugar, causing hot flashes. One of the biggest culprits is sugar. Sometimes just regulating sugar intake is enough to successfully control hot flashes.

Some of the other natural ways to alleviate severity and frequency of hot flashes include three to four hours of exercise per week, deep breathing and a healthy diet which includes plenty of the phytoestrogens-rich foods. Extensive research has also shown vitamin E—contained in whole grains, nuts and seeds, sweet potatoes and crab meat—can reduce hot flashes.

Stress is a major trigger in upsetting the balance in the body. Stress factors, such as busy schedules, emotional upsets and lack of adequate sleep and relaxation, all contribute to hot flashes. For a woman, looking after her emotional as well as physical needs is of paramount importance.

Infertility, Early Miscarriages and Post Natal Depression

All the above conditions relate to low progesterone levels.

According to Dr. Lee, "Estrogen dominance caused, once again, from progesterone deficiency has resulted in a near epidemic of infertility among women in their mid thirties. Excess estrogen seems to stimulate the ovaries to over-produce follicles, which, combined with delayed child bearing, results in an early burn out of follicles.

"I had a number of patients who had been unable to conceive. For two to four months I had them use natural progesterone from days 5 to 26 in the cycle (stopping on day 26 to bring on menstruation). Using the progesterone prior to ovulation effectively suppressed ovulation. After a few months of this, I had them stop progesterone use. If you still have follicles left, they seem to respond to a few months of suppression with enthusiasm and the successful maturation and release of an egg occurs. Some of my patients who had been trying to conceive for years had very good luck with this method. There are even few children named after me!"[7]

The chief cause of early loss of pregnancy is now thought to be luteal phase failure, in which ovarian production of progesterone fails to increase sufficiently during the first several weeks after fertilization. Maintaining the secretory endometrium (uterine lining) and the development of the embryo are dependent upon adequate luteal-supplied progesterone. The failure of progesterone production during this critical time of pregnancy mirrors the rising incidence of progesterone deficiency occurring ten or more years before menopause. Other contributing factors are stress, nutritional deficiencies and xeno estrogens.

When several miscarriages have occurred, Dr. Lee recommends progesterone supplementation (in addition to nutritional support), starting after ovulation (day 14 or so) and continued on after pregnancy is confirmed for an additional two months. After two months, placenta-driven progesterone becomes dominant. Reducing the supplemental progesterone during the third month should be gradual so as to avoid any abrupt drop in progesterone levels.[8]

As pregnancy advances, placental production of progesterone rises to a level of 350 to 400 milligrams a day (normally 20 milligrams) and the ovaries' contribution at that point is nil.

After delivery, the placenta-derived progesterone is suddenly gone. Since the adrenals are the primary source of progesterone at that time, if they are exhausted, there would be insufficient progesterone produced. Remember that progesterone is a natural anti-depressant.

Many women experience depression in the days and weeks following childbirth. Research by Brian Harris and his colleagues in Wales found that, among 120 women, those with the highest prenatal and lowest postnatal progesterone levels also scored highest on measures of post partum depression scores.[9]

Post partum depression is generally difficult to treat and often anti-depressants become the first line of defence. Natural progesterone would be a more sensible and safer approach.

Migraine Headaches

When migraine headaches occur with regularity in women only at premenstrual times, they are most likely due to estrogen dominance. Estrogen causes dilation of the blood vessels and thus contributes to the cause or causes of migraines. One of the many beneficial qualities of natural progesterone is that it helps restore vascular tone, counteracting the blood vessel dilation that causes headaches. Natural progesterone is certainly a more natural way to treat these migraines and avoids the need for more dangerous pharmaceutical drugs.

Ovarian Cysts

Ovarian cysts are products of failed or disordered ovulation. They may be asymptomatic or create pelvic pain. Some may grow to the size of a golf ball. Such cysts occur when, for reasons presently unknown, the ovulation did not proceed to completion.

To understand this cystic condition, it is essential to have an in-depth appreciation for the hormonal process. Each month one or more ovarian follicles are developed by the effects of follicle- stimulating hormone (FSH). Another hormone, luteinizing hormone (LH), is responsible for promoting ovulation and the transformation of the follicle (after ovulation) into the corpus luteum, the progesterone-producing structure. With each month's surge of LH, the follicular site swells and stretches the surface membrane, causing pain and possible bleeding at the site of the cyst.

The signalling mechanism that shuts off ovulation in one ovary each cycle is the production of progesterone in the other. If sufficient natural progesterone is supplemented prior to ovulation, LH levels are inhibited and both ovaries think the other one has ovulated, so regular ovulation does not occur.

Adding natural progesterone from day 10 to day 26 of the cycle suppresses LH and its luteinizing effects. Thus, the ovarian cyst will not be stimulated and, usually within a month or two, will regress and atrophy without further treatment.

Premenstrual Syndrome

PMS is identified by a collection of symptoms that usually occur one week to ten days before the menses. The most common symptoms include several or all of the following: bloating, weight gain, headache, backaches, irritability, depression, breast swelling or tenderness, loss of libido and fatigue. The full range of symptoms include confusion and disorientation, poor judgement and decision-making, mood swings, body aches, anger and verbal abuse, lethargy alternating with increased energy, alienation, guilt (at having abused friends), lack of self-esteem and cravings for sweets, especially chocolate. Further, every system in the body can be affected: immune, digestive, circulatory, nervous, endocrine and dermatologic (skin). Women experiencing PMS may experience any combination of the above and with varying degrees of severity, from mild to overwhelming.[11]

What is interesting to note about these symptoms is that they are the same as symptoms of estrogen dominance.

In his practice, Dr. Lee would measure the weight gain of his patients in the luteal phase of their cycle (the two weeks before the onset of menstruation). If he found that there was an increase in weight of three to six pounds at that time, he would conclude that the patient had PMS. The weight gain was the result of intracellular fluid retention (the swelling of all the cells in the body). The swelling of brain cells can result in the commonly reported PMS feelings of anger, irritability and hostility. Sound familiar? Natural progesterone also helps to alleviate these symptoms.

PMS is certainly an indication that there is significant hormonal imbalance occurring in the body.

Natural progesterone has proven to be highly effective when included in a regime for restoring hormonal balance. "In my practice, hundreds of women who were severely handicapped by PMS have been completely symptom-free with natural progesterone," reports Niels Lauersen, M.D., professor of obstetrics and gynecology at the New York Medical College. In his practice more than 90 percent of his patients who have tried natural progesterone have found relief.

Joel T. Hargraves, M.D., director of PMS and Menopause Clinics at Vanderbuilt University in Nashville, Tennessee, has also found impressive results using natural progesterone. "I've been using natural progesterone for 12 years and I haven't seen any long-term effects. It doesn't affect cholesterol levels, it doesn't affect Mother Nature—basically it is a wonderful thing."

A leading proponent of natural progesterone, Dr. Katarina Dalton has found that, "target cells containing progesterone receptors are widespread in the body, although most are found in the brain, particularly in the limbic area which is the area of emotion, rage and violence. The other receptor sites where progesterone should be received are the eyes, nose, throat, lungs, breast, liver, adrenals, uterus and vagina. All these are areas in which symptoms of PMS may occur such as headaches, asthma, laryngitis, pharyngitis, rhinitis, sinusitis, mastitis, alcohol intolerance and congestive dysmenorrhoea."[12]

While it is likely that a hormone imbalance directly or indirectly caused by progesterone deficiency is the major factor in the majority of PMS cases, there may also be other factors that deserve attention, especially in those cases that do not find complete relief with progesterone treatment. Contributing factors to PMS include poor nutrition as well as physical and emotional stress.

Sex Drive (Low Libido)

Sex drive, or libido, though mediated by sex hormones, is really a brain function. The underlying primary sexual drive in all mammals emanates from the brain centers mediated by sex hormones. The effect of progesterone on human libido has been largely ignored by mainstream medical research. The accepted belief is that estrogen is the primary sex drive hormone in women.

What is rarely understood is that the heightened sexual energy many women experience at the time of ovulation is the result of the surge of progesterone levels at the time of ovulation. Progesterone is the hormone necessary for increased libido, not estrogen as is commonly believed.

In studies with hamsters which had their ovaries removed, estrogen alone was insufficient to restore sexual receptivity; progesterone was required.[9] Dr. Lee reports that his patients' flagging libido returned only when progesterone was added. While testosterone is usually given the spot light as the key hormone for turning on libido, the role of progesterone is overlooked (remember that progesterone is the precursor of testosterone).

Skin Problems

When acne appears in women in their late thirties or forties, increased androgen (masculinizing hormone) is suspect. Dr. Lee has found that in almost all his female patients with this condition, supplemental progesterone cleared the skin. His hypothesis is that ovarian follicle depletion, leading to progesterone deficiency, results in increased adrenal production of androgens.

When progesterone is resupplied, androgen production goes down and the skin clears.

Seborrhea is a condition that causes flaking and itching skin without specific inflammation of the skin follicles. It, too, clears rapidly with topical progesterone cream.

Used as a skin cream, natural progesterone has a wonderful moisturizing effect on the skin. It increases hydration and oxygenation of the cells. Women using the cream have been impressed with the improved appearance of their skin. They have reported to me that wrinkles are disappearing! Natural progesterone has been an ingredient in moisturizing creams for the past 45 years.

Thyroid Deficiency

Thyroid is the hormone that regulates metabolic rate. Low thyroid tends to cause low energy levels, cold intolerance and weight gain. In his medical practice, Dr. Lee noticed that there were greater numbers of women taking thyroid supplements for hypothyroidism than men. He also recognized that many estrogen dominance symptoms, such as fat and water retention, breast swelling, headaches and low libido were present. When progesterone levels were increased, not only did their estrogen dominance symptoms decrease or disappear but so too did their presumed hypothyroidism.

Estrogen, progesterone and thyroid hormones are interrelated. Estrogen causes food calories to be stored as fat while thyroid hormone causes fat calories to be turned into usable energy. Thyroid hormone and estrogen have opposing actions. Dr. Lee has hypothesized that estrogen inhibits thyroid action in the cells creating hypothyroid symptoms despite normal serum levels of thyroid hormone. Symptoms of hypothyroidism occurring in his patients with unopposed estrogen (progesterone deficiency) lessened when progesterone was added and hormone balance was restored.[13]

Vaginitis, Vaginal Dryness and Thinning

There is a higher incidence of vaginitis in women taking the Pill, which often relates to the Pill's suppression of natural hormones. After menopause women are more predisposed to vaginal dryness as well as vaginal, urethral and urinary tract infections, although these are not inevitable consequences of menopause. Dr. Lee has noticed that, "Those who opted for natural progesterone therapy have been remarkably free of these problems. Further, their previous vaginal dryness and mucosal atrophy return to normal conditions after 3-4 months of progesterone use. Progesterone cream can also be used effectively and safely intravaginally. This suggests that natural progesterone also provides a direct benefit to vaginal and urethral tissues or may sensitize tissue receptors to the lowered levels of estrogens still present in post menopausal women."[14]

In addition, a diet rich in phytoestrogens is essential. Also, you can topically apply aloe vera gel or insert a vitamin E softgel capsule vaginally. (The pH of your body will break down the capsule so there is no need to puncture it.)

If, however, a more dramatic remedy is required, estriol cream (prescribed by your doctor) may help. A 1991 Norwegian review concluded that estriol is a safe, cheap and effective therapy for the symptoms of estrogen deficiency after menopause including atrophy of the vagina, uretha and bladder, urinary tract infections and abnormal function of the lower urinary tract. The researchers found that estriol had no metabolic effect or serious side effects at recommended doses and was safe for use long term.[15]

Chapter   **15**

Suggested Uses of Natural Progesterone

Natural progesterone, as stated earlier, is made from the Mexican Wild Yam. The most effective way to use natural progesterone products is absorption via the skin. Absorption through the skin is 40-70 percent more effective than ingestion. This is because the liver removes a high percentage of ingested hormones, returning them to the digestive tract where they are converted to water soluble forms that bind with other substances and are then eliminated from the body.

The most popular and effective progesterone products are available as creams, oils or roll-on's. In dermal transport, progesterone is first absorbed into the subcutaneous fat layer and then passively diffused throughout the body via the blood circulation. With continued use, fat levels of progesterone reach an equilibrium and successive doses of progesterone result in increased blood levels and stronger physiological effects. This is why progesterone applications may require two or three months of use before maximum benefits are experienced.

Every woman's body is unique. It is important for her to find the right dose for her body. The suggested dosages are merely guidelines. Women who are experiencing more severe symptoms may initially require larger or more frequent amounts. It is considered safe to experiment until the dose that is correct for your body is determined. It may also be necessary to try different products until the most desired results are experienced.

How to apply it?

Natural progesterone is most readily and easily absorbed by the thinner skinned areas of the body where there are plenty of capillaries. These include the areas where we tend to blush. The best areas are the face, neck, chest, abdomen and the upper and inner areas of the arm and thighs. Creams can be used as excellent moisturizers for the face. It is best to rotate the sites, applying cream to one area one day and another area the next day, etc.

When to use it ?

Application of natural progesterone follows the body's natural progesterone production. Since menstruation is the time of lowest levels of progesterone, it is advised that it not be used during this time. Application begins upon cessation of menstruation, which is usually day 8 of the menstrual cycle. Smaller amounts are applied two to three times daily for the next two weeks. During the last week of the menstrual cycle (day 21 to 28), the amount is increased, again following the body's own natural progesterone cycle. Depending on the concentration of progesterone in the product, 1/8 to 1/2 teaspoon is used per day, or 3 to 10 drops of oil. Roll-on application suggests an 8 inch strip once or twice daily. Be sure to follow the instructions that are provided with the product you are using.

If a woman no longer has periods, she can either follow the calendar month or count the day she begins as day one and apply natural progesterone for the next three weeks. It is advised to have one week off. However, some menopausal women find that they need to use the product daily in order to alleviate symptoms.

Hormone Replacement Therapy - How to Get Off It

Hormone Replacement Therapy is a combination of an estrogen and a progestin such as Provera. If a woman is taking both estrogen and a progestin, the first step is to substitute natural progesterone for the progestin, then gradually decrease the estrogen. Dr. Lee advises his patients to reduce the estrogen they are taking by 50 percent and to immediately stop using the progestin at the time they begin using natural progesterone. He has found no ill effects in stopping the progestin abruptly.

Then the next month they can reduce the estrogen again by 50 percent and the same for the next. By the end of the third month, the HRT can be safely and completely discontinued. Continue using the natural progesterone. It is recommended to use a 2 ounce jar a month over the three months. The cream can be applied for 21 days twice daily with a break of 7 days which will ensure that the hormone receptors are sufficiently stimulated. When a woman has successfully weaned herself off the HRT, she may then find that her body requires less cream.

When a woman on HRT wishes to stop taking it, there are a few things that need to be kept in mind. The first thing is that the progestins and natural progesterone compete for receptor sites in the body, so the full benefits of progesterone will be reduced until the progestins have been cleared from the body.

Secondly, blood levels of natural progesterone will not rise to optimum levels until 2 or 3 months after you begin to use the cream.

Thirdly, the use of natural progesterone cream may temporarily sensitize the estrogen receptors, leading to an experience of high estrogen effects—fluid retention, tenderness and swelling of the breasts, or even the appearance of scant vaginal bleeding. These are only temporary and will normally soon clear.

If a woman has had a hysterectomy and prescribed only an estrogen replacement, she can follow the same protocol as for weaning off of HRT, adding the natural progesterone and reducing her estrogen by half each month.

It is important to allow time for the levels of natural progesterone to reach physiological equilibrium as the synthetic hormones are reduced. Generally if the estrogen is stopped abruptly (and no natural progesterone is added) women will tend to experience symptoms of rapidly falling estrogen levels such as hot flashes, migraines and vaginal dryness. These symptoms are a form of withdrawal. It is not recommended to go 'cold turkey'.

If after three or four months, the natural progesterone does not eliminate all the symptoms, then Dr. Lee suggests that a woman may consider adding a little estrogen, usually in the form of estriol (the safest form of estrogen). However, most women report that the natural progesterone alone successfully addressed all their symptoms and were feeling better than ever.

Hysterectomies

Hysterectomies are the most common major non-obstetrical surgical procedure in the United States, second only to caesarean section. About 20 million American women have had their uteruses removed. Officially about 600,000 hysterectomies are performed annually. Unofficially, however, the figure is closer to one million. The average age at which women have this operation is 42. More than three-quarters of hysterectomies are performed on women under the age of 49. In fact, twice as many women in their 20's and 30's are hysterectomized as women in their 50's and 60's. It is estimated that fifty percent of American women will have a hysterectomy in their lifetime.

Dr. Stanley West, noted infertility specialist, Chief Of Reproductive Endocrinology at St. Vincent's Hospital, New York and author of The *Hysterectomy Hoax*, says, "more than 90 percent are unnecessary." He believes that, in general, a hysterectomy is never necessary unless a woman has cancer. Other more conservative views conclude that 50 to 90 per cent should not have been done. According to John Robbins in his best selling book *Reclaiming Our Health*, "What all the authorities agree upon is that 90 per cent of the procedures are elective, that there are alternatives in at least 90 percent of the cases, and that less than 10 per cent of the operations are in fact medically imperative."

Technically, a hysterectomy is the removal of the uterus and an oophorectomy or ovariectomy is the removal of the ovaries. Removal of the ovaries is also known in medical terminology as female castration. However, popular parlance now refers to the removal of the uterus and ovaries as a "total hysterectomy." Since women who have hysterectomies go into instant, surgically induced menopause, they are immediately put on estrogen replacement therapy (ERT) although estrogen (or any other drug or other treatments) will never successfully replace a woman's ovarian and uterine hormones or functions. Since estrogen has been implicated in endometrial cancer, only women without a uterus are now prescribed estrogen on its own without a progestin although estrogen still puts women at increased risk of breast cancer. Estrogen will also cause many women to experience all the ensuing estrogen dominant symptoms.

In whatever form it may occur, a hysterectomy is radical surgery for a woman. Women experience a loss of physical sexual sensation as a result. The procedure also tends to shorten, scar and dislocate a woman's vagina.

Some of the most common consequences, in addition to operative injuries are: heart disease, osteoporosis, bone, joint and muscle pain painful intercourse, displacement of bladder, bowel and other pelvic organs, urinary tract infections, chronic constipation and digestive disorders, short term memory loss, depression and dulling of emotions.

The leading reasons for recommending hysterectomies are fibroids (usually the cause of heavy bleeding), endometriosis, and uterine prolapse (the uterus falls from its normal position). Fibroids and endometriosis respond extremely well to natural progesterone cream as well as dietary and other nutritional support. A prolapsed uterus, in addition to following dietary and nutritional guidelines, has been successfully treated with naturopathy, Traditional Chinese Medicine and other natural healing modalities. Obviously, a woman has a right to be informed of these effective and much less invasive alternative treatments.

Usually women with hysterectomies are told by their doctors that they must remain on estrogen for the rest of their lives. However, this is not true. Dr. Lee has his patients wean themselves off the synthetic hormones by gradually reducing the dosage (following the same protocol as described for coming off HRT). In those very few women who still have hot flashes or vaginal dryness, he gives them some estrogen cream, usually estriol to use intravaginally for a few months. They are then able to taper off the estriol completely. Natural progesterone combined with a good diet, exercise, appropriate nutritional support and stress management will insure women who have had hysterectomies as well as oophorectomies renewed hormonal balance without ever needing synthetic hormones.

Menopause

All women experience menopause differently. Some women's bodies require higher progesterone levels than others. The correct amount for one woman is not necessarily the right amount for another. The cream can be applied according to the calendar month and applied over a 14 to 21 day time period. Then discontinue application until the next month.

For vaginal dryness or discomfort, the cream can be applied intravaginally. This may be in addition to or instead of your daily applications.

If hot flashes or night sweats are severe, women have found relief by applying the cream every fifteen minutes for the next hour following the episode.

Some women find that they require increased amounts of cream daily to find relief from their symptoms. These women may need to use the cream for the entire month rather than taking 7 days off.

When progesterone levels are increased, estrogen receptors become more sensitive—that is, they are more likely to respond to estrogen. Thus, some women notice that after a week or two of applying progesterone, some vaginal bleeding may occur due to their own estrogen levels. At that point, a woman may stop the progesterone for a week or two and then start again for a three week period.

During the week while being off of the progesterone, there may be some bleeding. This is due to the persistence of estrogen production, which will diminish over time. This is the advantage of stopping progesterone for one week each month. It allows the estrogen-induced blood buildup to be shed.

In cases of persistent spotting or vaginal bleeding (for more than three months), consult your physician.

Osteoporosis

Three of the best methods to accurately determine the degree of bone loss in osteoporosis are serial dual photon absorptiometry (DPA), dual energy x-ray absorptiometry (DEXA) and ultrasound densitometry. These tests measure bone density very precisely, are relatively low in cost and emit minimal radiation. It is suggested that, if possible, you have one of these tests done before you begin using the cream in order to establish a base line from which to measure changes in bone density. Subsequent tests may be performed at six month or one year intervals so you and your physician can monitor bone growth, however testing is not mandatory to begin using the cream.

For people with mild osteoporosis or for prevention of osteoporosis, follow the general recommendations for the natural progesterone. If you have severe osteoporosis or have experienced fractures, the daily amounts can be increased up to 1/2 teaspoon per day. Follow the suggested schedule of three weeks on and one week off (during the time of menstruation, if applicable).

Peri-menopause

Peri-menopausal women often experience the signs and symptoms of estrogen dominance. These include water retention, headaches or migraines, fatigue, breast swelling, fibrocystic breasts, depression or mood swings, loss of sex drive, heavy or irregular menses, uterine fibroids, cravings for sweets, weight gain (particularly around the hips or thighs) and low thyroid symptoms of cold hands and feet.

A peri-menopausal woman can follow the generally recommended dosage of natural progesterone. What appears to be the onset of early menopause is often discovered to be estrogen dominance. As progesterone levels increase, the estrogen dominant symptoms will disappear. There is a tendency for doctors to prescribe estrogen if irregular bleeding occurs, however there is no reason to give estrogen if there is still menstrual bleeding. Menstrual bleeding indicates that there is no estrogen deficiency. Irregular menstrual periods may be the result of low progesterone levels. If you have been put on estrogen for irregular periods, taper down the estrogen and begin using the suggested guidelines for natural progesterone.

It is recommended to use the cream approximately two weeks per month. Between day 12 and day 26 to approximate normal progesterone levels. Some women with longer cycles can take it from day 10 to day 28. If bleeding starts before day 26 (or before it would normally begin), stop using the progesterone. You can then resume using it on day 12. It may take three cycles before normal periods are achieved.

When migraine headaches occur premenstrually, estrogen dominance is often a contributing factor since estrogen dilates the blood vessels. Normal vascular tone is able to restored by using natural progesterone. Natural progesterone can be used ten days before the onset of menstruation. Dr. Lee suggests applying 1/4 to 1/2 teaspoon every three to four hours until the symptoms subside. This usually only necessitates one or two extra applications. He also advises that higher doses of progesterone can be quickly attained with sublingual drops which are more rapidly absorbed than skin cream.

PMS

To use for PMS, follow the above recommendations. However, if you experience cramping or other symptoms during menstruation, you may apply the cream until the symptoms dissipate. The cream can be rubbed on to the lower abdomen during menstrual cramping. If you have migraines during your cycles, the cream can be rubbed on to the back of your neck or on your temples.

As time goes by and the symptoms diminish, try cutting back each month on the amount of natural progesterone you use. If symptoms return, resume the previous dosage. Ultimately, your goal is to be hormonally balanced and symptom free. If you have no symptoms for several months and then symptoms recur, you may want to use the cream as needed. The best way to know if enough is being used is if your symptoms are relieved.

Chapter 16

Natural Estrogens—The Good Guys

Specific plants contain compounds that mimic the actions of estrogen or that favorably affect estrogen metabolism in some way. Although they are considered to be extremely weak compared with human hormones, when used in the diet or in specific natural remedies, they can alleviate menopausal symptoms.

These plant derived estrogens, known as phytoestrogens, are present in a wide variety of foods and herbs. If a woman has an excessive amount of estrogen, these substances help to block the estrogen from entering the estrogen receptor sites. If there is not enough estrogen, they fill the gap. When beneficial phytoestrogens bind to receptor sites, they can not only supply an alternative form of natural estrogen where needed but by taking up estrogen sites, they may protect the woman from environmental xeno-estrogens which are continually trying to key into those sites.

Phytoestrogens appear to block the effects of excess estrogen stimulation in organs such as the breast and uterus and well may be protective. A particularly rich source of phytoestrogens is found in soy products such as tofu, tempeh, soya milk and miso. One study of Japanese women suggested that a high intake of these products was the reason why they had so few hot flashes or other menopausal symptoms as well as low rates of breast cancer.

An incomplete list of other foods rich in phytoestrogens includes cashews, peanuts, oats, corn, wheat, apples, almonds, rye, lentils, French beans and pomegranates. Obviously it is essential to eat a diet rich in these foods.

Phytoestrogens have been a part of natural remedies for women's hormonal problems for hundreds of years, if not longer. Herbs used in women's formulas included black cohosh, alfalfa, licorice, red clover and sage. Black cohosh has been known to be a popular herb used by the Native Americans for female complaints.

Estriol - The Underestimated Estrogen

Estriol, along with progesterone, is the estrogen that is made in large quantities during pregnancy. It is made by the placenta. These two main pregnancy sex hormones have potential protective properties against the production of cancerous cells. Estradiol, on the other hand is 1,000 times more potent on breast tissue than estriol. It is well documented that overexposure to estradiol, and to a lesser extent estrone, increases a woman's risk of breast cancer, whereas estriol is protective.[1]

An important 1966 *Journal of American Medical Association* article by H.M. Lemon, M.D., reported a study showing that higher levels of estriol in the body correlate with remission of breast cancer. He showed that women with breast cancer had reduced urinary excretion of estriol. He also observed that women without breast cancer have naturally high levels of estriol and that these women are at much lower risk of breast cancer than other women. Estriol's anti-cancer effect is due to its ability to block the stimulating effects of the other estrogens by blocking the estrogen receptor sites on breast cells.[2]

In fact, A. H. Follingstad, M.D., presented results in *The New England Journal of Medicine* of a study in which small doses of estriol were given to a group of post-menopausal women with spreading breast cancer. An impressive 37 percent of them experienced a remission or arrest of their metatastic lesions. There have been reports that it is better than tamoxifen for women with breast cancer.[3]

Estriol is the estrogen most beneficial to the vagina, cervix and vulva. In cases of post-menopausal vaginal dryness and atrophy which predisposes a woman to vanities and cystitis, estriol supplementation would be the most effective and safest estrogen to use. It is also an effective treatment for urinary tract infections.[4]

In addition, estriol, has benefits similar to that of the stronger estrogens but without the risks. It not only reduces menopausal symptoms but increases cardiac function with improved blood flow to the extremities.

Estriol treatment also results in the re-emergence of friendly lactobacilli bacteria and the near elimination of pathologic colon bacteria.

While estriol offers so many benefits to women's health, like natural progesterone, it cannot be patented. It already has established an excellent safety record through its proven track record in Europe as both a prescription drug and an over-the-counter product. Once again, the influence of the pharmaceutical companies and the reluctance of doctors to investigate safe alternatives, restricts a woman's safe and effective options.

While HRT is generally recommended to provide a source of estrogen for women after having a hysterectomy, natural herbal remedies containing phytoestrogens herbs as well as supplementation with estriol, in addition to natural progesterone, can provide adequate levels of hormones, making HRT unnecessary. If a woman has been eating a healthy diet with abundant amounts of phytoestrogen-rich foods, there is usually adequate estrogen available to her from other estrogen sites in her body such as body fat. After a hysterectomy, it is always advisable to receive advice and guidance from health professionals. Contrary to popular opinion, however, a hysterectomy does not automatically mean a woman must go on HRT for the rest of her life.

Chapter 17

The Relationship Between Hormonal Imbalance and Disease

Exposing the Myths

HRT is now almost universally recommended to menopausal women for a wide variety of reasons. The most significant reasons women are encouraged to embark upon the HRT band wagon are HRT's supposed contribution in preventing or lessening the effects of osteoporosis, cardio-vascular disease and more recently, Alzheimer's disease. The tremendous fear of these illnesses that is instilled in patients by well-meaning doctors who, after all, are the targets of effective pharmaceutical advertising and education (usually the only source of information they receive about these products) often over-rides a woman's natural instincts. It's time to unravel the myths that hide the real story.

Osteoporosis

Dr. John Lee, writes the following about the myths of osteoporosis:

Osteoporosis Myth #1—
Osteoporosis is a calcium deficiency disease.

Most women with osteoporosis are getting plenty of calcium in their diet. It is quite easy to get the minimum daily requirement of calcium in even a relatively poor diet. The truth is that osteoporosis is a disease of excessive calcium loss caused by many factors. In osteoporosis, calcium is being lost from the bones faster than it is being added, regardless of how much calcium a woman consumes.

Osteoporosis Myth #2—
Osteoporosis is an estrogen deficiency disease.

Not even basic medical texts agree with this—it is a fabrication of the pharmaceutical industry with no scientific evidence to support it. Osteoporosis begins long before estrogen levels fall and accelerates for a few years at menopause. Taking estrogen can slow bone loss for those few years, but its effect wears off within a few years after menopause. Most importantly, estrogen cannot rebuild new bone.

Osteoporosis Myth #3—
Osteoporosis is a disease of menopause.

This is at least a decade short of the truth. Osteoporosis begins anywhere from five to 20 years prior to menopause when estrogen levels are still high. Osteoporosis accelerates at menopause or when a woman's ovaries are surgically removed or become non-functional, such as can happen after a hysterectomy. It is staggering to think how many thousands or millions of women have been doomed to a crippled old age and early death because their ovaries and/or uterus were unnecessarily removed before menopause and natural progesterone replacement ignored.

To understand osteoporosis it is important to know a bit about bones. Bone forming cells are of two different kinds. One type are called osteoclasts and their job is to travel through the bone in search of old bone that is in need of renewal. Osteoclasts dissolve bone and leave behind tiny unfilled spaces. Osteoblasts move into these spaces in order to build new bone. A lack of estrogen as experienced at menopause indirectly stimulates the growth of osteoclasts, increasing the risk for developing osteoporosis. HRT containing estrogen should therefore help prevent osteoporosis. From this point of view, it does.

While osteoclast cells have been shown to have estrogen receptor sites, osteoblast cells, which are responsible for making new bone, have been shown to have, not estrogen, but progesterone receptors. What this means is that it is progesterone (the natural form, not the synthetic progestins) not estrogen which is responsible for building bone tissue.

This view is upheld in *Scientific American's* updated medicine report text, 1991, which states, "Estrogens decrease bone resorption but associated with the decrease in bone resorption is a decrease in bone formation. Therefore, estrogen should not be expected to increase bone mass." The authors also discuss estrogen's side effects, including the risk of endometrial cancer which "is increased six-fold in women who receive estrogen therapy for up to five years; the risk is increased to 15-fold in long term users". So, while estrogen has been shown to slow bone loss in women, it does not arrest it and, in fact, can contribute to other serious health problems.

Slowing down bone loss is in no way the same as building up bone mass. Not only does the use of estrogen for osteoporosis have only a partial effect but what effect it does have is not necessarily permanent. One group of researchers found that within four years of discontinuing estrogen, there was no detectable difference in bone mineral content between women who had never taken the drug and those who began treatment but gave it up. Other studies have shown that six years into menopause estrogen may stop being effective.[1, 2]

Dr. Kitty Little from Oxford found masses of tiny clots in the bones of rabbits treated with hormones. She is convinced that HRT, in the form of estrogen and progestins, will increase the risk of osteoporosis. Blood clots originate from sticky clumps of platelet cells in the blood. She believes that blood clots in the bones can cause bone to break down, leading to osteoporosis.[3]

The early studies on which the estrogen-protection assumptions were based had gross scientific defects. Dr. Jerilynn C. Prior, and her colleagues, reporting in the *New England Journal of Medicine*, confirmed that estrogen's role in combating osteoporosis is only a minor one. In their studies of female athletes, they found that osteoporosis occurs to the degree that they become progesterone deficient, even though their estrogen levels seemed to remain normal.[4]

Dr. Prior continued her research with non-athletic women. They showed the same results. While both these groups of women were menstruating, they had anovulatory cycles and were, therefore, progesterone deficient. Dr. Prior then went on to discover that anovulation and a short phase cycle now occurs in up to 50 percent of North American women's menstrual cycles during the final reproductive years. Unfortunately these major findings went relatively unnoticed in the medical community.

As a result of her extensive review of published scientific evidence in this area, Dr. Prior confirmed that it is not estrogen but progesterone which is the bone tropic hormone—that is, the bone builder. They were even able to identify progesterone receptor sites on osteoblast cells (bone tissue building cells). Nobody has ever found osteoblast receptors for estrogen. The bottom line is that it is in women with progesterone deficiency that bone loss occurs.[5]

More and more research findings are emerging that challenge the estrogen deficiency/osteoporosis relationship and reinforce the progesterone deficiency link. The results from a three year study of 63 post-menopausal women with osteoporosis verify this. Women using transdermal progesterone cream experienced an average 7-8 percent bone mass density increase in the first year, 4-5 percent the second year and 3-4 percent the third year. Untreated women in this age category typically lose 1.5 percent bone mass density per year! These results have not been found with any other form of hormone replacement therapy or dietary supplementation.[6]

Dr. Margaret Smith, a specialist in medical gynecology and medical founder of the first menopause clinic in Western Australia, believes that, "In the next five years we are going to find that natural progesterone is going to replace or displace all the progestins because it will be shown to be that much more effective in actually restoring bone loss, not just preventing bone loss, as well as making women feel well."

Despite this clear evidence of the importance of progesterone to bone formation, very little attention has been given to it by the medical establishment. Dr. William Regelson, a leading researcher in hormones and the author of *The Super-Hormone Promise*, flatly states, " Given the fact that 25 percent of all women are at risk of developing osteoporosis, I think it is unconscionable that progesterone's role in this disease has been neglected."[7]

Another intriguing fact sheds serious doubt on estrogen's key role in bone health. Studies using tamoxifen which is an anti-estrogen drug given to breast cancer prone women to block the uptake of estrogen hormones have shown no bone loss in women. If lack of estrogen is the cause of osteoporosis, tamoxifen would have caused significant bone density loss.[8]

Bone loss is the result of many other factors besides progesterone deficiency. Excess protein in the form of meat and dairy products (contrary to the dairy industry's advertising) contribute to bone loss. An acidic condition is created in the blood which then causes the body to extract calcium from the bones to neutralize it. Another major factor is lack of exercise. Bone growth is dependent on weight bearing exercise. In addition, sugar, diuretics, antibiotics, inadequate levels of hydrochloric acid in the stomach, caffeine, fluoride, cigarettes, alcohol abuse and cortisone all are deleterious to bones.

There is a huge amount of confusion about the place of calcium supplements as a safeguard against osteoporosis. It seems, in fact, that calcium supplements are raising some concern. *Lunar News* (December 1994) reported, "it is unclear why the risk of hip fracture is doubled by high calcium." Another study showed that calcium supplementation in adults, normal elderly subjects or the osteoporotic, had little effect (less than 4 percent increase) on bones, but it did increase constipation and flatulence (more than 10 percent).[9]

The best source of calcium is from calcium-rich foods which include sardines, canned salmon, dark green leafy vegetables, Brazil nuts, tofu and all soy products, sunflower seeds and hulled sesame seeds.

In summary, post menopausal osteoporosis is a disease of excess bone loss caused primarily by a progesterone deficiency and secondarily by poor diet, nutritional deficiencies and lack of adequate weight bearing exercise. While progesterone assists in the restoration of bone mass and is an essential factor in the prevention and proper treatment of osteoporosis at any age, it should be considered as one of several key ingredients in bone health.[10]   Bone building is a chain of linked factors each of which must be strong for the chain to be strong.

Cardiovascular Disease

Estrogen is being touted by mainstream medicine as a great preventive of cardiovascular disease in women and therefore a major reason to have women on HRT. To understand the issues at hand, it is first important to understand just what is cardiovascular disease. Cardiovascular disease incudes both heart disease and stroke. Stroke, like heart disease, is a vascular disease: a disease of blood vessels. In both cases the blood vessels become narrow either through spasm or through atherosclerosis, the narrowing of the arteries that feed the heart. Therefore not enough blood gets to a critical place. In the case of heart disease it is the heart and with strokes it is to the brain. Cardiovascular disease also encompasses high blood pressure and coronary artery disease.

Dr. Susan Love says, "Heart disease is not a symptom of menopause. Heart disease is heart disease. It's more common in postmenopausal women that in pre-menopausal women but that's because postmenopausal women are older than pre-menopausal women. It's like gray hair; you're more likely to have gray hair after menopause than before it but menopause doesn't cause gray hair - rather, they both tend to happen in later life.

"The standard line has always been that women are

protected from heart disease as long as their bodies make estrogen, and then after menopause they lose that protection and
the rates of heart disease for men and women become equal.
But in fact, the rates never become equal. In this country,
women in their sixties and seventies have 45 per cent less heart
disease than men in the same age bracket. Women develop
heart disease much later than men - seven or eight years later.
Women's risk rises continuously as they get older but there's
no sudden increase with menopause. We never catch up."[11]

It is interesting to note that the *Physician's' Desk Reference*
warns that women should not take estrogen or progestins if
they have current or past clotting disorders, thrombosis, a
stroke history, cerebrovascular or cardiovascular disorders,
high lipoproteins (a specific type of blood fats), severe uncon-
trolled hypertension or lipid metabolism disorders. In addition, cigarette smoking increases the risk of serious cardiovascular effects from the use of estrogens.

It is also an undisputed fact that estrogen and progestins,
the two key ingredients of oral contraceptives, have been responsible for strokes, blood clots and heart attacks in women
taking The Pill. There is presently a class action suit underway
in the UK by women who claim that HRT caused their strokes
and blood clots.

Estrogen does appear to lower total cholesterol and raise
HDL cholesterol (the good one) modestly. However, it is no
where conclusive that this reduces the risk of heart mortality
per se. Significant new findings also show that natural progesterone has the same effect.

In light of these known risks, it is certainly curious that
estrogen and the use of HRT is so rigorously pursued by the
pharmaceutical companies and the medical profession as a
treatment for the prevention of cardiovascular disease.

According to Dr. Lee, the one notable study which formed the entire basis of the positive estrogen-cardiovascular link, the 1991 *New England Journal of Medicine* report known as the *Boston Nurses' Questionnaire Study* (conducted using a large sampling of nurses), was radically flawed and the statistics manipulated.[12] Although there is ample evidence from numerous other studies showing that, indeed, the opposite is true—estrogen is a significant factor in creating heart disease—these findings have been virtually ignored in the frenzy for profits. Dr. Lee goes on to say that pharmaceutical advertisements neglected to mention the fact that stroke death incidence from that study was 50 percent higher among the estrogen users.

In 1985, another notable study, the Framingham Heart Study, the only ongoing, long-term epidemiological study in the United States conducted on 240,000 women reported that their postmenopausal estrogen users had 50 per cent more heart disease and twice as much cerebrovascular disease as non-users. Estrogen users had a higher risk of vascular disease which was independent of other main known risks such as early menopause.[13] Their conclusion was that there is no coronary benefit from estrogen use. In fact, other studies have found increased cardiovascular disease risk from estrogen use. In her *New England Journal of Medicine* letter to editor, following the publication of the *Boston Nurses Questionnaire Study*, Dr. Jerilynn C. Prior listed 16 references disputing the claim that estrogen provided cardiovascular benefit.

Alarming evidence has recently surfaced from animal studies which demonstrates that synthetic progestins (Provera) co-administered with estrogen, counteracts any beneficial effects estrogen may have in preventing heart disease and stroke.

It actually was found to increase the risk of coronary vasospasms, narrowing of arteries to the heart that can lead to a heart attack.[14]

While researching the estrogen-cardiovascular link Nancy Beckham found the following:[15]

* High doses of estrogens are likely to be thrombogenic (blood clotting) during use and it is possible that even moderate doses may increase the risk of clotting among women who smoke or who already have clogged arteries. Reports are now starting to come in indicating that high-dose estrogens, particularly as experienced with estradiol implants, cause hyper-coagulability, which means that the blood has a tendency to clot, thereby increasing the risk of heart attacks and stroke.

*A British medical report also states that the cardiovascular effects of synthetic progestins used with estrogen in the much larger number of women who have not undergone hysterectomy are unknown.

* Some researchers do not consider that heart disease is linked to the cessation of the body's estrogen production. (Actually it is inaccurate to use the word 'cessation' since estrogen production is only reduced in menopause.)

Natural progesterone seems to play a significant role in protecting women from cardiovascular disease. We know now that anovulatory cycles and lowered progesterone levels occur prior to menopause; and progesterone levels after menopause are close to zero. Estrogen, on the other hand, falls only 40-60 percent with menopause. A woman's passage through menopause results in a greater loss of progesterone than of estrogen. Perhaps the increased risk of heart disease after menopause is due more to progesterone deficiency than to estrogen deficiency. Dr. Lee has noted in his clinical experience that lipid profiles improve when progesterone is supplemented.[16]

In an interview published by the American Medical Association on the Internet, Dr. Elizabeth Barrett-Connor remarked, "If I were treating a woman primarily because she had dyslipidemia (abnormal blood fats) and low NDL cholesterol, I would probably see if she wanted to take micronized progesterone. I was quite impressed with the better effect." What is known about progesterone is that it increases the burning of fats for energy and has an anti-inflammatory effect. Both of these actions could be protective against coronary heart disease. Progesterone protects the integrity and function of cell membranes, whereas estrogen allows the influx of sodium and water while allowing the loss of potassium and magnesium. Progesterone, a natural diuretic, promotes better sleep patterns and helps lessen stress. When one reviews the known actions of progesterone, it is clear that many of its actions are also beneficial to the heart.

When it comes to increased risks of coronary disease, dietary factors are extremely important. Heart disease risk is increased by the following: general overeating, animal fats, sugars and refined carbohydrates, over processed foods, excess salt or sodium, trans fatty acids, lack of fibre, magnesium and/or potassium deficiency and lack of anti-oxidant rich food or supplements such as vitamins C, E, A, beta-carotene, folate and selenium. Stress is also a risk factor for heart disease.

Cardiovascular disease would be much more effectively treated if more attention was placed on its many contributing factors. According to Dr. Graham Colditz, Harvard professor and project director of the *Boston Nurses Questionnaire Study* the known breast cancer risk for women from estrogen is of such concern that other more effective treatment and life style approaches should be the first line of defence. They include: stop smoking, exercise, Vitamin E and folate, weight reduction and dietary changes.

The observations of Dr. Elizabeth Barret-Connor were written in a paper in 1993. She stated, "No other prescription drug has been given on such a large scale to prevent disease in healthy women without proof of efficacy by a randomized clinical trial .... It is also important to remember that estrogen replacement is drug treatment, not really replacement therapy; the dose and route are unphysiologic and the level of circulating estrone is higher than sustained by pre-menopausal women."[17]

Hormones and Cancer

The evidence connecting female cancers of the breast, uterus and ovaries with high estrogen levels is growing. Estrogen's job in the uterus is to cause proliferation of the cells. Under the influence of estrogen, uterine cells multiply faster, then progesterone normally should be released at ovulation and stop the cells from multiplying. Progesterone causes the cells to mature and enter the secretory phase that causes the maturing of the uterine lining, which is now ready to receive a possible fertilized egg. Estrogen is the hormone that stimulates cell proliferation and progesterone is the hormone that stops growth and stimulates ripening.

Breast Cancer

Estrogen dominance also stimulates breast tissue: premenstrual women who suffer from estrogen dominance often suffer from breast swelling and tenderness. Progesterone, as a hormone of maturation, brings the cells back into balance and thus can eliminate breast tenderness.

There is certainly an alarmingly high incidence of breast and uterine cancer amongst western women. There is evidence that breast cancer occurs most often at the stage of life when estrogen is dominant for the full month and progesterone is not coming in ovulation—the halfway point. Dr. Graham Colditz, maintains that the use of unopposed estrogen for 10 years or more is responsible for 30-40 percent of breast cancers. However, women who took estrogen plus progesterone increased their risk by up to 100 percent[18]

Johns Hopkins Private Obstetrics and Gynecology Clinic accumulated 40 years of research which was published in the *American Journal of Epidemiology* in 1981.[19] What they discovered was that when the low progesterone group was compared to the normal progesterone group, it was found that the occurrence of breast cancer was 5.4 times greater in the women in the low progesterone group. That is, the incidence of breast cancer in the low progesterone group was over 80 percent greater than in the normal progesterone group.

When the study looked at the low progesterone group for all types of cancer, they found that women in the low progesterone group experienced a tenfold increase from all malignant cancers, compared to the normal progesterone group. This would suggest that having a normal level of progesterone protected women from nine-tenths of all cancers that might otherwise have occurred. It is interesting to note that the study disappeared into oblivion when there was no money available to pursue the obvious implications of a progesterone deficiency role in cancer.

In a 1995 study published in the *Journal of Fertility and Sterility*, researchers did a double-blind randomized study examining the use of topical progesterone cream and/or topical estrogen in regard to breast cell growth. The result showed that women using progesterone had dramatically reduced cell multiplication rates compared to the women using either the placebo or estrogen. The women using only estrogen had significantly higher cell multiplication rates than any of the other groups, The women using a combination of progesterone and estrogen were closer to the placebo group.[20]

This exciting study provides some of the first direct evidence that estradiol significantly increases breast cell growth and that progesterone impressively decreases cell proliferation rates, even when estrogen is also supplemented.

It has also been shown that among premenopausal women, breast cancer recurrence or late metastases after mastectomy, was more common when surgery had been performed during the menstrual cycle, when estrogen is the dominant hormone, than when surgery had been performed during the progesterone dominant latter half of the menstrual cycle.

Recently there have been disturbing studies about still another possible effect of hormone therapy on the risk of breast cancer. This has to do with the effects of HRT on breast tissue. HRT can stimulate breast tissue causing it to become more dense. Cancer and breast tissue are the same density, so a mammogram can give false readings. Researchers at the University of Washington looked at the records of 8,779 postmenopausal women who had mammograms for breast cancer. Women on estrogen had 33 percent more false positives (showing an abnormality but none could be found) and 423 percent more false negatives (an abnormality was missed that showed up later) than women not using estrogen.[21]

Tamoxifen - Beware

At this point, it is important to explore the implications of the experimental drug tamoxifen, a synthetic hormone similar in structure to DES which has been prescribed to more than three million women with breast cancer since 1970. Since it is purported to have anti-estrogenic effects it is used as a breast cancer treatment, blocking the uptake of estradiol and estrone (the cell proliferating estrogens) and thereby protecting the breast tissue from the cancer-promoting estrogens present in the body. Among the choices of orthodox medicine, it certainly is the kinder treatment compared with chemotherapy, radiotherapy or surgery.

However, tamoxifen is not without its dangers. It is a known carcinogen. One study showed that 27 percent of women taking tamoxifen showed hyperplastic (unfavorable new growth) changes in their wombs within fifteen months.[22] Taking 20mg of tamoxifen per day can increase the risk of developing uterine cancer by up to five times.

In addition, eye damage, retinopathy, has been reported in seven per cent of women in one study, while menopausal symptoms such as hot flashes, vaginal discharge or dryness, irregular menses, nausea and depression are the most common side-effects. Thrombo-embolic disease (a clotting disorder) is seven times more frequent. According to Dr. Susan Love when it's taken for a year, tamoxifen increases bone loss in premenopausal women though it does prevent further bone loss in postmenopausal women.

Dr. Susan Love also reports that, "there is reason to believe that even tamoxifen's supposed role in preventing breast cancer should be questioned. Earlier studies had shown that when women who had cancer in one breast took tamoxifen, it reduced the risk of cancer in the other breast by 30-50 per cent. A more recent randomized controlled study, however, showed that it had its maximum effect with women who took it for five years. Taking it for five more years didn't offer any more protection and may actually have caused more cancers, In other words, after a while the breast cells become resistant to tamoxifen and actually start to be fed by it."[23]

One study showed just a meagre 0.7 percent benefit for women taking Tamoxifen preventively to reduce the risk of developing further tumors in the breast.[24] To make matters worse, Dr. Ellen Grant, author of *Sexual Chemistry*, has reported that in tamoxifen treated subjects, new tumors that do appear tend to be highly malignant with an increased mortality.

While a known carcinogen, the *Science News* (March 2, 1996) reported rather shocking information about Tamoxifen. The World Health Organization (WHO) has formally designated tamoxifen as a human carcinogen, grouping it with roughly 70 other chemicals, about one-quarter of them pharmaceuticals that have received this dubious distinction.[25]

However, there are safer alternatives to tamoxifen. One of the estrogens produced by the ovaries is called estriol (weaker than the other two, estradiol and estrone). Estriol is considered a safe estrogen in that it has been shown to inhibit breast cancer. Dr. Henry Lemon and his colleagues conducted a study in women who already had breast cancer that had spread to other areas of the body. One group was given estriol and another not.

At the end of the study, 37 percent of those women who received estriol had either a remission or an arrest of their cancer.[26] Might not estriol, a natural, safe hormone with almost no side effects, be able to accomplish what Tamoxifen does but without the toxic side-effects?

A growing number of doctors also insist that the same results can be achieved by giving natural progesterone.

It is also interesting to note that menstruating women who have breast surgery carried out during the second half of their menstrual cycle—the luteal phase when progesterone is high to balance estrogens —survive far longer than do women whose surgery is done early in their cycle, during the estrogen-dominant follicular phase.[27]

Endometrial Cancer

The only known cause of endometrial cancer is unopposed estrogen. Here again the culprits are estradiol and estrone. Estrogen supplements given to post menopausal women for five years increase the risk of endometrial cancer sixfold and longer-term use increases it 15-fold. In peri-menopausal women, endometrial cancer is extremely rare except during the five to ten years before menopause when estrogen dominance is common.[28]

Cervical Cancer

Synthetic hormones are also linked to cervical cancer. The cells of the cervix are extremely hormone-sensitive. Levels of synthetic progestins, low enough not to alter the cells of the lining of the womb, have been shown to change the cells that line the cervix. Progestins dry up cervical secretions and this may be part of the reason why cancer of the cervix develops quickly in the presence of cervical infections.[29]

Ovarian Cancer

On May 1, 1995, the American Cancer Society announced further alarming statistics from a study of ERT and ovarian cancer. It showed that among the 240,000 post-menopausal women who had no prior history of cancer, hysterectomy or ovarian surgery. Participating in this 13 year prospective mortality study, the risk of fatal ovarian cancer was 40 percent higher for women who used estrogen for at least 6 years and 70 percent higher at 11 years of use. The obvious conclusion from the study was that long-term use of estrogen replacement therapy may increase the risk of fatal ovarian cancer.[30]

Melanomas

It was predicted in the 1960's that the Pill would increase the chances of a woman developing a melanoma, the most lethal of all skin cancers. Hormones control the pigmentation of our skin and melanoma cancer cells have estrogen receptors which can make the growth of cancer more likely. Women taking the Pill and HRT are at greater risk in developing melanomas than the average woman.

In animal tests, estrogen stimulates the formation of the

black pigment melanin but the effect is greatly augmented by the addition of a progestin - as in the Pill. Because hormones control pigmentation, the early researchers thought that oral contraceptives would predispose to the development of malignant melanomas.[31] The tumors, like breast cancer cells have estrogen receptors and women on HRT are also more likely to develop melanomas.

The Walnut Creek study found Pill and HRT users were more likely to develop melanomas. All the women who developed melanomas under age forty had taken the Pill. By 1981, the overall increased risk for ever-users was statistically significant at three times.[32]

An Australian case-control study described how more than five years of pill use significantly increased the melanoma risk if the pill had been started ten years before the cancer was diagnosed. The increase remained significant even after adjustment for many factors. The study found increases among women who had been given hormones to regulate their periods, as HRT or to suppress lactation.[33]

Alzheimer's Disease

Just the mention of Alzheimer's strikes fear in the heart of people. Nothing seems to be as devastating as the loss of mental faculties. While the medical profession has given Alzheimers's disease a rather high profile these days, it actually isn't all that common. It is also more likely to affect the very old. It's 14 times more common in people over the age of 85 than in those between 60 and 65 years of age. It seems that women have 1.5 to 3 times more risk of getting Alzheimer's than men which may, in part, simply be because women live longer.[34]

A theory has been suggested that estrogen may protect against Alzheimer's disease. As is so often the case with synthetic hormones, an hypothesis has been quickly transformed into unsubstantiated fact.

The study that gave credence to this theory was published in the *American Journal of Epidemiology* in 1994. The study was based upon a group of 127 postmenopausal residents in a retirement community in California called Leisure World. Investigators compared the women whose death certificates mentioned Alzheimer's or dementia with the matched record of decedents who hadn't died of either cause. They found that estrogen users were 30 percent less likely than non-users to have died of either condition. The researchers also found that Alzheimer's patients on estrogen performed better on a standard mental exam than patients who weren't.[35] The researchers of the study believe that it hints at a possible connection but research is far from conclusive.

It is important to remember that in the world of medical research and clinical trials there are usually conflicting data and results. So, it comes as no surprise that in a quite similar study involving residents of Rancho Bernardo, California, women decedents who had taken estrogen were found to be almost twice as likely to have died of Alzheimer's disease as women who had never taken it. Further, when the researchers compared the test scores for memory and mental acuity of the users and never-users, no significant differences were found.[36]

While inconclusive as well as conflicting results about the estrogen-Alzheimer link compete for medical and public attention, the pharmaceutical companies along with medical establishment are jumping the gun on estrogen's benefits on the brain. Dr. Love reported that one of Ayeth-Wyerst's representatives (the manufacture of Premarin) announced at a conference on hormones that "cognition can provide the gut-level response to breast cancer." The implication was that if the makers of Premarin could show that estrogen prevents Alzheimer's disease, it would be enough of a benefit to counteract women's fear of getting breast cancer from taking estrogen: fear of Alzheimer's trumps fear of breast cancer.[37]

Once again, sensational advertising campaigns can successfully masquerade as factual medical science.

Chapter　18

Men and Natural Progesterone

It seems that men can also benefit from natural progesterone. In men, progesterone is synthesized by their testes to produce testosterone and in their adrenals to produce corticosteroids. Healthy men continue to produce normal testosterone and corticosteroid levels into their seventies and eighties.

A common treatment for men with prostate cancer is to castrate them either chemically or surgically in order to lower their testosterone levels. It is believed that prostate cancer growth is slowed when testosterone is reduced. As a result of the rather abrupt reduction and in some cases where there was almost a complete absence of testosterone, a kind of male menopause is induced. Hot flushes are not uncommon. A lack of testosterone will accelerate bone loss within a year or so resulting in osteoporosis. Testosterone, in a similar fashion to progesterone, is able to stimulate new bone growth thus increasing bone density.

Dr. John Lee has found that, "If one wishes to prevent or treat the castration-induced osteoporosis, it is possible to safely supplement progesterone to replace testosterone in these men."[1]

A personal account from a contributing doctor to the guidebook *Alternative Medicine: The Definitive Guide* confirms a similar experience. "Topical application of natural progesterone may prove beneficial in the treatment of prostate conditions. The doctor reports working with twelve men, all in their late seventies, who were suffering from osteoporosis. As it has been well established that natural progesterone applied topically, can relieve osteoporosis, the physician suggested that the men systematically massage it into their skin on a daily basis. All of them began to experience relief from their condition and later called to tell (the doctor) that, after three months, they were also experiencing an improved urine flow, with less pressure on their prostate glands and noticeable decrease in nightly urination."[2]

Dr. Norman Shealey, medical practitioner and author, also believed that natural progesterone benefits men. He began to use natural progesterone on his older male patients. The progesterone apparently caused one patient's DHEA hormone level to double. His libido soared and he felt better than he had in years. In fact. Dr. Shealey discovered that the majority of men who used the natural progesterone cream showed a marked increase (60 to 100 percent) in their DHEA. This is important news, since DHEA seems to spark the metabolism of both men and women and helps balance the entire glandular system. More research on the connection between these two hormones is definitely in order.[3]

Chapter 19

An Integrative Approach

There are a number of ways in which women can attend to the various symptoms and illnesses that hormonal imbalance may be causing. Dietary changes, exercise, naturopathy, chiropractic care, classical osteopathy, Chinese herbs and acupuncture, homeopathic and herbal remedies, aromatherapy and stress management techniques are some of the safe and effective options presently available. There isn't necessarily just one way. Having the options to integrate more than one therapy into a woman's preferred choice of treatment provides her with the best of each modality. Doctors and complementary health practitioners both have their place in a woman's health care. Ideally, working in partnership with a woman's needs would provide her with the most successful outcome.

Chapter 20

The Challenge Before Us

The hormone story is certainly a very complicated one. Up until now only one version of the story has been available to the majority of western women. Serious doubt has been cast on the efficacy and appropriateness of estrogen and progestins as the first choice in treatment. Women are certainly suffering more than ever before from a wide variety of female complaints. What complicates the hormone story is that the seeming cures for these complaints may actually make them worse. Without understanding the far-reaching side-effects of estrogen dominance and progestins, doctors are often mis-diagnosing the cause of these aggravated conditions. Other drugs may then be prescribed, with disastrous effects, as the spiral of unnecessary medication increases. What is the toll being taken not only to a woman's deteriorating health and emotional well-being but also to her financial situation, her relationships and her career?

Without adequate knowledge, education and access to natural products, women have been easy prey to the powerful campaigns of the multinational drug companies that have convinced doctors and governments of their claims. It is becoming more evident that women's interests are not always best met through such a biased approach. It is not unusual for profits to take precedence over health and well-being. The last thing a woman needs is to have her natural bodily functions denigrated to deficiency diseases which then necessitate ongoing medical attention

The long road we have been travelling for almost 40 years has encouraged and promoted the wide range of synthetic hormone products and it is taking us to a tragic dead-end. The scare tactic techniques and intimidation employed by doctors and pharmaceutical companies alike to use such products, often over riding a women's better judgment, have pushed millions of women into using drugs that are unproven and unsafe. It is no surprise, therefore, that Dr. Lee has issued an ominous warning when he says, "we will soon regard making estrogen the key ingredient in Hormone Replacement Therapy as a major medical mistake."[1] Unfortunately, the same can now be said about progestins.

The same message is reiterated by Leslie Kenton in her book *Passage to Power* when she says that "one of the greatest ironies at the turn of the millennium is that for almost half a century women have been encouraged to use estrogens. They have been sold as a means of birth control and for counteracting negative symptoms experienced at menopause. Yet it turns out that excessive estrogen may well be the greatest enemy any woman in the industrialized world ever faces."

Women must be able to make educated, informed choices about their bodies and their health treatment preferences. It's impossible to make important health decisions if fundamental facts are missing or misconstrued. It is also evident that the health care providers we have come to rely upon either have not received adequate, unbiased education themselves or have become imprisoned by their own arrogant and narrow-minded points of view.

According to Dr. Lee, "There is revolution underfoot. The revolution is not driven by doctors. The revolution is being driven by the women. There is probably no better teacher for doctors than a resourceful, assertive, intelligent woman who knows what she is talking about. When she goes to her doctor and says, 'I have tried estrogen, it made me bloat, it made my breasts swell, it made me feel terrible and I couldn't concentrate (and a whole long list of other side-effects) so I decided to go on the progesterone cream and reduce my estrogen and now I am so much better. I want you to follow me in this', remembering that this is the way to carry on the revolution."

It is indeed time for women to take even greater responsibility for their health, their choices and their life-style. The greatest weapon against compliance and ignorance is knowledge. It's time to ask poignant questions of your health provider, to demand answers and to be willing to investigate safe, alternative approaches. It is apparent that women will need to participate in educating their doctors of the other choices that exist as well as the ones that they prefer. It is a woman's right to choose with dignity the best approach to her own health care.

It is up to every woman to read, question, trust her natural instincts and learn about her own body. It is also essential that women honor their own cyclic nature and intuitive wisdom. A woman's body is her ally in her search for health and healing. Listening to the wisdom of her body is the path to self-discovery, joy and well-being.

Recommended Reading:

Dr. Susan Love's Hormone Book, Dr. Susan Love,
Random House

Estrogen & Breast Cancer, Carol Ann Rinzler,
Hunter House, Inc.,

Hormone Replacement Therapy: Yes or No, Ketty Kamen, Ph.D.,
Nutrition Encounter

Menopause and Estrogen, Ellen Brown and Lynn Walker,
Frog, Ltd., California

Passage To Power, Leslie Kenton,
Random House

Reclaiming Our Health, John Robbins,
H J Kramer, Inc.

The Menopause Industry, Sandra Coney,
Spinnifex Press

What Your Doctor May Not Tell You About Menopause,
Dr. John R. Lee, Warner Books

Women's Bodies, Women's Wisdom, Dr. Christiane Northrup,
Bantam Books

Part Two —

The Journey to Hell and Back

Women's Personal Stories

A Personal Perspective -

In writing this book, it was first a journey of researching the facts. I sifted through piles of articles, journals, studies and books. As part of this academic exercise, I personally tracked down and interviewed the experts for their opinions on the subject. It was a massive learning experience. I uncovered startling research that seriously challenged the zealous promotion of synthetic hormones' supposed wonders. (Studies that somehow disappeared into oblivion.) I also learned how statistics have been tinkered with and manipulated to give credence to any theory or point of view. Medicine has always been, after all, a battle field for competing hypotheses that rise and fall out of favor on a regular basis. However, facts and stats, as enlightening as they may be, are still intellectual abstractions devoid of the flesh and blood of human experience.

This book would have been a glorious intellectual exercise if it wasn't for the intimate experiences I had while talking with hundreds and hundreds of women. They spoke of their confusion, physical and emotional pain, despair and anger. It was as though they had become lost in an endless maze of doctors' visits, tests and medications. A maze that always led to another dead end. They also spoke of how their HRT experience shattered self-esteem, relationships and careers. And that horrible helplessness feeling that comes when you know your health is mysteriously draining away accompanied by the terror when your bodily functions seem to be careening completely out of control.

The following personal journeys are authentic stories from women who unknowingly found their lives to be casualties of synthetic hormones found either in oral contraceptives or HRT. They bravely consented to share their personal experiences as testimonies to the courage, inner wisdom and perseverance that eventually brought them back to health. Their stories are truly inspirational. While they may seem extreme, in fact, women all over the world have been recounting similar experiences. I have heard thousands of variations of the same theme. These are women who were fortunate to find their way out of the synthetic hormone induced darkness. Their collective wish is that their experiences may serve as beacons of light guiding other women safely on their way to greater hormonal health.

Kate's Story

As a 38 year old mother of three, I began to experience hot flushes and cessation of my period two years ago. All the signs indicated early menopause so I promptly consulted a specialist physician who heads a local menopause clinic for women. She prescribed oral estrogen (Premarin) and when this failed to raise my serum levels, she suggested Estraderm patches then finally an estrogen and testosterone implant. Synthetic progestin (Provera) was taken orally from day 14 to 26.

It struck me, while bracing myself against the pain as my GP cut a small incision in my backside, that I'd have to subject myself to this implant procedure every six months for the rest of my life in fear of heart disease or osteoporosis. Without question, pharmaceutical-driven propaganda had successfully convinced me that menopause was indeed a disease and that I could not survive my life cycles without medical intervention.

Ill health had plagued me since the birth of my third child and a tubal ligation in March, 1989. Diffused muscle soreness and stiffness was diagnosed as fibromyalgia that had become so chronic I lived on 2-3 Mercyndol a day. Excessive weight gain (40 lbs.) and loss of energy did little for my libido. Bloating, sleep disturbance, chronic fatigue, incontinence, tender and somewhat lob-sided breasts and migraines all intensified over time. My face became dry and pimply with the added bonus of excessive facial hair.

HRT was introduced to alleviate symptoms, protect against early aging and restore my health.

At no time did I understand exactly (1) why I was on HRT other than it was recommended in the treatment of menopause,

(2) what quantifiable gains I could expect or (3) the risks involved.

My inner disquiet spilled over into my relationship with family and friends. I made other people miserable because that's how I felt within myself. I'd become downright aggressive, exhibiting dramatic mood swings that usually ended in a teary apology. Some days the anxiety attacks were so severe I'd climb into bed, pull the covers over my head and wouldn't come up for air all day. Getting through the day was a major feat. I was spiralling down a black hole that swallowed me by degrees every day. And what I feared most was the loss of my loved ones as my growing madness was mirrored in their eyes.

Of course, I tried pouring my heart out to a psychologist but quickly realized he did little more than pull on an already depleted bank account. Certainly, I knew I wasn't insane. It just felt that way most of the time.

May 1996, in preparation for an implant, I was injected with a high dose of estrogen. Even before my physician had removed the syringe, my breasts were stinging. The sensation was not unlike that of a mother's breast filling or 'letting down' with milk during breast-feeding. My GP reassured me it wasn't anything to be concerned about. I figured if she wasn't concerned then everything must be ok! We were both wrong. Four months later a second opinion confirmed a lump in my right breast.

Since offering my body up to HRT over an eighteen month period, I was hospitalized for tests to investigate vaginal bleeding that included a D&C, repair of cervical erosion and cancer screening of the cervix, uterus and breast. Why was my physician so vigilant for cancer? Did HRT involve risks I'd not heard about?

One day, I some how got my tablets mixed up. I mistook a

few Premarin tablets for Provera and overdosed on estrogen. My body, already weakened in its struggle with the estrogen implant, could not handle the introduction of this extra estrogen. And what followed made a miscarriage look rather tame. Fifteen days later and still clotting, my doctor prescribed synthetic progestin every two hours until the bleeding came back under control. After this episode of heavy bleeding, I began to seriously contemplate a hysterectomy.

On the assumption my symptoms were directly the result of too much estrogen in my body, I decided to try a Natural Progesterone cream. I began massaging the cream onto my face, arms, tummy but concentrating on my breasts. Some weeks later, after cancelling my mammogram appointment three times, I finally found the courage to front up for tests. To my utter relief, the results came back all clear. Remarkably, there was no lump to investigate. And if that wasn't irrefutable evidence of the positive effects from natural progesterone, I also began menstruating again naturally.

Initially my menstrual flow was heavy with excessive clotting. Nonetheless, over a matter of months my period took on a regular, more natural cycle. Natural Progesterone appeared to have a positive impact on estrogen's known side effect - thickening of the endometrium.

These days I'm up out of bed around 5:00 am most mornings and rarely do I reach for a Panadol. I no longer suffer from fibromyalgia, incontinence or fibrocystic breasts. My energy levels and libido have returned and my weight has stabilized. For the first time in my reproductive life I can chart my menstrual cycle on a calendar!

Whatever my condition one thing is for certain, Natural Progesterone restored my health where prescription drugs could not. I concluded that the much publicized HRT debate is not about what the doctors or pharmaceutical companies claim will or should work in my body. It's about making an informed choice and having access to ALL the facts and remedies, both orthodox and complementary. After all, I am the walking, talking laboratory animal on whom these drugs are tested.

Franka's Story

As I look back at the last twelve years of my life, I can only but give thanks that I am still alive today. At 51 years of age and a psychologist with a successful practice, I am only now beginning to recover my physical and psychological health from my descent into the hell that HRT caused me. Of course, for all that time I had no idea that the very hormone drugs I was being prescribed were actually responsible for my deteriorating condition.

It all began at the age of 38 when I became aware of increasing hot flashes, leg cramps, dizziness and extreme mood swings. My GP diagnosed me as having an early menopause and prescribed Premarin. I stayed on that medication for the next six years.

However, over that time my symptoms continued to worsen. My gynecologist at that time decided to change my medication to 1.25 mg. of Ogen with Provera for tens days of the month. I was told to take three tablets of Ogen daily. For a brief time I thought the HRT was working as my hot flashes, leg cramps and mood swings seemed to stabilize. But it was only temporary and before very long my symptoms and a whole host of others returned with a vengeance.

My emotions would seesaw from violent outbursts of anger and rage to uncontrollable weeping. I became increasingly more depressed and anxious, finding myself obsessing with worry over the smallest things. I had found myself transformed from a very positive and optimistic person to one who had to struggle to find anything good in a situation. I was getting more and more critical, especially with my family members. I fought with my daughter, actually coming to blows with her once - something that I had never done my whole life. My life really descended to the depths when I decided to separate from my husband of over twenty years. I was constantly critical and angry with him. He could do nothing right in my eyes. Through all this, my self-esteem was eroding away.

Riding this extreme roller coaster of emotions made me feel as though I was possessed. At the time, I didn't put any of these symptoms down to the HRT, I just thought that I was going crazy. My GP recommended anti-depressants and suggested psychiatric help for my rages. So, I followed his advice and began seeing a psychiatrist.

Besides the emotional turmoil, I was suffering with daily migraines that would begin in the afternoon and continue until I went to sleep at night. In addition to the migraines, I also had insomnia for which I was prescribed sleeping tablets.

Then there were the sore breasts that were so painful at times I couldn't even buckle my seat belt. The litany of complaints continued with severe bloating, frequent urination, extreme fatigue (diagnosed as chronic fatigue), worsening eye sight, dizzy spells that were with me on and off for ten years, reduced sex drive, dry and aging skin, increased blood pressure, food sensitivities, chronic constipation, aches and pains throughout my body, dry and lifeless hair and skin so sensitive that if I was touched it felt raw and exposed. I felt premenstrual all the time. I was once a fit athlete but now my muscle strength had deteriorated to such an extent that I could hardly lift my briefcase.

What added to my despair was discovering that my teeth had lost 50 - 70 percent of their bone density. All my doctors' warnings that without HRT I would become a victim to the ravages of osteoporosis were proven absurd since my excessive bone loss coincided with the increased use of HRT.

I'm sure that if I wasn't such a strong person I would have certainly attempted suicide. There were times when my life seemed like such a nightmare that I wished I just wouldn't wake up in the morning. The worst part was the fear that my life was careening totally out of my control.

Throughout the years, I made endless visits to doctors...gynecologists, neurologists, opthamologists, internists and psychiatrists. I spent thousands of dollars on office visits, tests and medications without benefiting one iota. Not once during all those years, did any doctor ever suggest that HRT could be behind all these symptoms. In fact, I was told that I would have to remain on estrogen for the rest of my life.

From a once healthy, vital, athletic, positive person, I had become devoid of energy, health and self-esteem. Even my once alert and active mind had deserted me. I felt as though I had rapidly arrived at old age. I was convinced that I was dying as all the life energy seemed to be sucked from me. I prayed for a miracle.

The miracle arrived in the form of a friend insisting that I read some information about estrogen dominance, the side-effects of HRT and the benefits of natural progesterone. Since my health felt so delicately balanced on a precipice, I was scared and confused about any kind of change. It took me some time before I was able to gather the courage to try this new avenue.

My first decisive step was to cut my Ogen from 3 tablets to 1 1/2. I literally went cold turkey for six weeks enduring incredible withdrawal symptoms which included an extreme feeling of being disconnected from myself, aches and pains, sadness, sweats, and dizziness to the point of almost passing out . My resolve paid off, however, when after that time my migraines ceased as did my dizziness. I then began to use a transdermal cream of natural progesterone. I know it sounds incredible, but within ten minutes I started to giggle (a rare experience for me at that time) and my mood lifted and I felt as though I had emerged from a fog. After four days my energy began to return and my bloating started to go down.

I also began to see a holistic doctor who was informed about estrogen dominance and natural alternatives. He verified my condition as estrogen dominant. His diagnostic tests showed that my toxicity levels were so high that they were equal to someone who had cancer! It was an understatement to say that my body was a mess! No wonder why I had felt so crazy. I committed to his program of detoxification, dietary changes, nutritional support and natural progesterone cream.

It is now three months since I first began using the cream. My energy increases daily. My anger has disappeared entirely and I'm feeling "up" ninety-five per cent of the time. I'm sleeping more soundly now and reducing my sleeping tablets. My mind is clear and sharp and my intuition is flowing again. My dry and itching skin is retuning to its earlier softness. Even the wrinkles are fading! My digestion is improving and I am no longer bloated. My husband and I are living happily together once again and I'm so grateful for all his infinite patience, loyalty and understanding.

All the years I was on HRT were as though I was living a zombie existence and now, at long last, I have finally returned to the land of the living! I now find myself laughing and enjoying life more than I ever did before. There is no doubt in my mind that HRT was the cause of all the symptoms, physically and emotionally, that plagued me during all those years. My anger at being abused by the medical profession has transformed into a burning passion to get the message out to as many women as possible about the dangers, risks as well as safe alternatives to HRT.

I have grown immensely from this intense period of my

life. I learned that menopause can be a really positive and empowering change in a woman's life. I now live everyday filled not only with an overflowing gratitude for everything and everyone but with a new and profound appreciation for myself as a woman.

Terri's Story

At 27 years of age, I was experiencing hot flashes and really bad night sweats. In addition I was tired all the time, had insomnia, headaches, aching hands, an aching neck, mild depression and no sex drive. I first noticed these symptoms, especially the hot flashes, four years ago. However, at that time my GP assured me that there was nothing to worry about.

Since my symptoms continued to get worse my GP did another series of tests. This time the tests showed that my estrogen levels were low. He pointed the finger at stress. Since I was working long hours, gruelling hours at a stressful job as a TV producer as well as enjoying a rather active social time, I thought it was all starting to catch up with me. I decided to take time off to take care of myself and did nothing but rest and sleep.

When my symptoms continued, I was referred to an endocrinologist who suggested that I may be going through an early menopause, discussed the possibility of going on to an IVF program and sent me off to do a battery of tests over the next six weeks. She also immediately took me off the Pill which I had been on continuously since I was fifteen years old (which I now believe was a major contributing factor in my long history of hormonal imbalance).

When all the test results were in, the specialist announced that even though she didn't exactly know what my problem was, she decided to prescribe HRT for me anyway and told me to chart my symptoms. I began taking a half of .625 mg. of Ogen. When I asked her about the possible side-effects, she told me not to worry about it and sent me on my way.

After a short time, my hot flashes were reduced but my headaches increased to three time or more a week, I was constantly fatigued and generally felt unwell.

For more than a year I stayed on the HRT. When my hot flashes and night sweats returned, I sought out several other opinions but the answers were all the same. I had early menopause and was told, in fact, to increase the dose of HRT. Within a year I was taking two tablets of .625 mg. Ogen daily.

I was now feeling absolutely terrible. I was unable to work for a year. My motivation was gone as was my self-esteem. I was totally exhausted, continued to have regular headaches, hot flashes, no sex drive and aching neck and hands. I became so depressed that I was further prescribed anti-depressants.

By this time, I was really concerned about my ability to have a child so I investigated an IVF program. In order to evaluate my hormone levels, I was told to go off my HRT. When I expressed my concern about going cold turkey, the nurse said I would "just have to handle it."

It was a nightmare. Going cold turkey gave me debilitating migraines. I had intense hot flashes every five minutes and such bad night sweats that I didn't sleep for five nights. I sank deeper into depression assuming that the increase in symptoms meant that my health was deteriorating. I was never warned that the HRT was addictive and that by not taking HRT I could be plunged into instant withdrawals. It never dawned on me that I was a "estrogenaholic".

In the darkest depths of my despair, I chanced upon information explaining the effects of estrogen dominance. I immediately recognized all my symptoms! I sought out a holistic doctor who confirmed my suspicions. I was diagnosed with estrogen dominance. He also said that my liver was damaged due to the toxic effects of the Pill. He immediately began to wean me off of HRT with a natural progesterone cream, changed my diet (eliminating dairy, sugar and wheat while increasing vegetables, fruits and grains) and began a detoxifying program.

After two months on this program, I am now feeling wonderful. My headaches are gone along with my depression. For the first time in over a year I'm excited again with the prospect of going back to work. I have energy in abundance and all my aches and pains have disappeared, My hot flashes and night sweats are almost gone. The most exciting news is that my doctor promises me that my body will be totally rebalanced within a year and that I will be fit and healthy to conceive a child.

I have just turned 29 years old, and I feel like I have finally gotten my life back. I also realize that I was misdiagnosed and misprescribed from the beginning. I was never going through an early menopause. The combination of the Pill and stress certainly triggered my earlier symptoms. I know now that it was the high dose of estrogen in combination with the synthetic progestins in the HRT that really sent my health and emotional well being plummeting into the worst time of my life. I trusted all the experts who really hadn't a clue about what was wrong with me and therefore actually contributed to making the problem much worse.

If I hadn't come across the information about estrogen dominance and found a sympathetic, holistic doctor, I shudder to think what would have happened to me, physically and emotionally. I was certainly heading for big trouble. I'm finally learning to listen to the wisdom of my body and to find the safest and most natural approaches to restore harmony. I have also learned in a very personal way that my health is the most precious thing I have. Without it, nothing else really matters.

Linda's Story

I began using the Pill at the age of seventeen at the insistence of my father . Even though I wasn't sexually active at the time, he, no doubt, thought he was doing the right thing by encouraging me to take preventative measures. I went off the Pill for a year, then back on again for another two years before taking another year's break. I resumed the Pill four years ago at the age of 24 when I entered a committed relationship. During that "on and off" time I didn't particularly notice any symptoms but then again I was young and wasn't aware of those sorts of things.

Two years ago, I began to notice a number of symptoms that were affecting my body and mind. Symptoms that could be categorized as PMS became progressively more severe. I became very bloated with my stomach protruding out and becoming very hard. There was also excessive fluid retention. My breasts and nipples were becoming so sore and painful that I couldn't stand to get hugged. I also was now getting really intense cramps at the beginning of my period. They would be so severe that all I could do was lie in a fetal position in bed during the first day of my period until they subsided. My periods were becoming heavier and I would have a discharge for several days after they finished. I also discovered noticeable hair growth....those dark, thick kind. They were appearing on different parts of my body - my jaw line, between my breast and even on my big toes! My head hair, however, was falling out. Mentally my thinking was really foggy around ovulation time. I would inevitably make unnecessary mistakes at work at that time.

The long list of symptoms continued. My libido disappeared " big time". Floating, sparkling flecks would often appear as though swimming in my field of vision. I have a family history of varicose veins and while on the Pill they appeared and became quite prominent. I experienced excruciating pains in my lower back on the day my period began. I felt like I just wanted to bend my body all the way over backwards to alleviate the pain. There was also the weight gain of more than seven pounds.

What really started to weak havoc with my life, however, were the emotional outbursts. I became extremely critical of everyone and everything, especially myself. I would find myself picking on my partner for the smallest thing which would always wind up in a fight. About two weeks before my period I would transform into the most angry, irrational person. There were times when I could hardly contain the rage and other times when I would fall into a heap and burst into tears for no apparent reason. These symptoms became more extreme with each month. At first I would have these PMS symptoms two weeks out of the month, then three weeks and then it seemed as though I was in a perpetual state of PMS. My life became a living hell. My life was totally out of my control and I felt terrified as though I were completely possessed by unwanted demonic forces .

Throughout those years of physical and emotional pain, my partner's unconditional support and love helped me through the most difficult of times. He was the one who would often recognize that my symptoms were hormonally related. He was usually much more aware of my monthly cyclic changes and their Jeckyl and Hyde effect on me.

I was disappointed, to say the least, that during the entire time I was on the Pill I was never given adequate information from doctors. Although I was once warned of the risk of strokes and blood clots from the Pill, none of its side-effects nor its other potential dangers were ever mentioned. Certainly the Pill was never mentioned at all as a possible cause for my symptoms.

In desperation, I began using a transdermal natural progesterone cream. It took me a little while to really get serious about using it. When I finally committed in the second month to the twice daily application, positive changes began to happen. My breast tenderness stopped completely as did the bloating and fluid retention. I no longer had cramps nor heavy bleeding. The lower back pain disappeared. My thinking became alert again, as though a fog had lifted. And even my libido made its return debut !!! Most incredibly, my emotional life came back into balance. I no longer felt irritable and negative. I began to feel beautiful within myself once again! Instead of lethargically moping around the house with a rather unkempt, grubby appearance, I suddenly was motivated to look after myself and my appearance again. My self-esteem emerged as though awakening from the Pill's spell.

All these changes occurred while I was using the natural progesterone cream even though I was still on the Pill. I also made dietary changes as well as paying more attention to my cyclic wisdom, charting my menstrual cycles and tuning into the moon etc.

As I became more aware of myself as a woman, it became obvious to me that the Pill was no longer appropriate. About four months ago, I decided to stop taking it altogether. I'm still in the process of balancing out my body after it's intense assault from all those years on the synthetic hormones. I'm also eating more healthily, learning to take more time for myself and consulting with a Chinese Herbalist. My physical and emotional health has improved immensely and am aware that I am now walking a path not only of greater hormonal balance but also personal power.

Sally's Story

I went through a comparatively early menopause in my mid-forties. The shock of my mother's unexpected death seemed to trigger my symptoms. Within a very short time I was experiencing night sweats (though no hot flashes) in addition to other medical problems brought on through grief.

At that time I was not seeing a gynecologist and didn't pay much notice to my symptoms. It was only when I went to a woman's clinic for a routine mammogram (I have a family history of breast cancer) that I mentioned my symptoms to an attending doctor.

After a consultation I was put on an HRT with estrogen pills. I was told that I would feel marvellous and " back to normal" (what ever that is). I tried a number of different brands trying to find one that suited my body. None made me feel well or, in fact, better in any way. In addition I was now bloated and having headaches which I now suspect was exaggerated by the progestin, Primulut.

When I tried to use patches, I discovered I was allergic to the adhesive backing which caused me to break out in water blisters.

I was, therefore, advised to try implants. In addition to a full implant of estrogen, I also was given a 50 percent strength implant of testosterone - the latter supposedly to give energy and impetus to carry on my business life. When I had the first of these, I immediately felt much better very quickly. I had this initial rush of euphoria accompanied with lots of energy and improved sleep . After a couple of weeks, things settled down. The only problem was an increase in fluid retention which seemed to all settle in my buttocks and thighs. I was advised to have a new implant every six months.

However, as the initial benefits began to wear off, I felt like a clock rapidly "winding down". To counteract this problem I decided to put myself onto a timetable of a new implant every four months. There was never a problem about having it done so frequently since no doctor ever questioned my decision nor asked me to have a blood test to determine the level of estrogen in my blood.

It was only at my sister's instigation and insistence that I finally went to see her gynecologist. The doctor insisted on a blood test before she would give me my requested new implant. The results showed that my estrogen level was extremely high. Despite this result, I was desperately needing a "fix".

My doctor refused to give me another implant until my levels had become normal. For the following 18 months I had a monthly blood test to monitor the levels. Each month she refused until she was happy with the results.

Of course, when she refused to give me another implant I was forced to go off "cold turkey". I didn't realize at the time how addictive implants were nor was I prepared for how shocking I would feel. The withdrawal symptoms included extreme fatigue, loss of energy and an accompanying lack of enthusiasm for life. My sleeplessness also returned.

Finally, when my levels were sufficiently reduced, I received another implant. This time it was only estrogen since I was concerned about the testosterone I had been absorbing into my body. What bliss! Within a couple of days, I was on another high!

However, by now I was starting to question where I was going and what was happening to my body. I was really uncomfortable with estrogen's effect on my weight gain which went from 126 lbs. to about 135 lbs. My clothes no longer fit so I gave about half of my wardrobe away. I was tired of people commenting on how much weight I had gained. It was apparent to me that as long as I stayed on the estrogen there was nothing I could do to lose the extra pounds. It became more and more obvious to me that this wasn't what my body wanted.

After being introduced to information about the symptoms and dangers of estrogen excess and its addictive nature, I immediately identified myself as having a dependency on the implants—a little like a heroin junkie. Since I used to be a heavy smoker, I knew how difficult it can be to break an addiction. I was concerned that my addictive tendencies would keep me hooked on my implant.

To cut a long story short, I completely stopped using HRT. Once again I went cold turkey but this time with the help of natural progesterone cream. One year on I feel so much better. My breasts are less sore and less lumpy. My energy level has improved and my weight is getting back to normal. The fluid retention has disappeared and my attitude toward life is once again enthusiastic. I have since been trying out a number of natural progesterone products to find out which one suits me the best.

I have been extremely lucky that through all my problems from the initial symptoms through to the withdrawals some years later, I have had the never ending consideration and love of my husband. Without his support and care, I don't know what would have happened.

Last November, my gynecologists found a lump deep in my left breast—the one that had been "lumpy" on the side for some time. This lump was in the middle of the breast. A breast surgeon scheduled a biopsy a month later. Fortunately for me the lump was benign. It was a condition known as radial scar. In conversation with my surgeon, she commented that she was seeing more and more women with breast lumps of various kinds in the years since HRT had become popular. She said that since she was approaching her menopausal years, she decided never to take HRT because of its implication with an increased risk of breast cancer.

I have personally persuaded many women, both friends and acquaintances, to stop using HRT and to consider a more natural approach such as including soy products in their diet and using natural progesterone cream. I'm once again like the zealous reformed smoker I was many years ago! Since giving up HRT my body is on the mend. I now find myself wanting to inform as many women as possible about the safe and natural alternatives to HRT so they can potentially avoid serious health problems in the future.

Part Three —

The Feminine
Path to Power

Chapter 1

Nostradamus' Predictions

Four hundred years ago, Nostradamus, perhaps the most famous of all visionaries, foresaw that the end of this millennium would usher in an unprecedented period of history when the influence of the feminine would transform all of society. His powerful predictions announced the end of the patriarchal order which has so dominated the course of history for the past five thousand years. This predicted ascendancy of the feminine will be responsible for not only initiating a massive experience of human renewal but also a completely new vision of how all of life can be an expression of harmony.

Included in his prophecies was the prediction that medical science would find ways of healing the body through formerly misunderstood natural cycles. He went on to reveal how the balance of hormones in a woman connects her with and aligns her to the earth's rhythms. Returning to the understanding of a woman's cyclic nature will restore the magic of the feminine and the wisdom of her instinctual nature. Nostradamus believed that only by such a transformation could humanity's survival be assured.

So, as the end of the millennium looms near, a massive awakening of women is required to fulfil the promise of Nostradamus' inspirational vision. Never before in history have so many millions of women sacrificed their hormonal balance, thus themselves, into the embrace of medical science. Besides creating devastating health problems which are only now coming to light, synthetic hormones have so altered a woman's natural rhythms that her powerful connection to her inner sense of Self has been seriously compromised.

What would it be like to know that in the deepest depths of your being as a woman, every part of your anatomy and each process of your female body contained ancient wisdom, a well-spring of creativity and unfathomable power?

As we welcome a new millennium, it appears that women are also welcoming a new sense of Self. The essential nature of a woman is cyclical, expressed by her monthly flow of changing hormones, energies and emotions. Life is about recurring cycles. It is expressed in the changing rhythms of the moon and the seasons. It is also found in the cosmic cycles described by the ancient sciences of astrology and numerology. The return of the feminine and women's awakening to a deeper appreciation of themselves is part of a greater cycle.

Chapter   2

Forgotten History

Extensive archeological research has now verified that beginning approximately 38,000 years ago humanity worshipped the feminine principle personified in the symbolism of the Goddess.

From Old Europe through Greece, Egypt, the Near East, India and the Far East, the Great Goddess was perceived as an organizing principle of the universe who embodied all the forces of life, death and rebirth within her figure. Her dominion encompassed not only the human world but also the plant and animal realms, earth and heaven and the seasonal and sky cycles. The Goddess was the embodiment of the life force that animated all of existence.

The Goddess religions embraced the constant and periodic renewal of life in which death was not separate from life. This religion displayed a deep respect for the natural cycles of women. In the societies where she was worshipped, women held exalted roles as priestesses, leaders, healers, midwives and diviners. These cultures held a deep reverence for the earth as the giver of life. The female form represented the embodiment of the power of nature.

Noting the correlation of the twenty nine days for the moon cycle with the twenty nine days of women's menstrual cycles, the ancients surmised the moon must be feminine. The rhythm of the moon, whose phases resonated to women's menstrual cycles, held a special place in the myths, religion and symbols of the Goddess. The Goddess teachings held that death was but the precursor to rebirth and that sex could be used not only for procreation but also for ecstasy, healing, regeneration and spiritual illumination.

Archeological remains from these cultures show no evidence of fortifications, weapons or violent deaths from warring. For tens of thousands of years these Goddess-oriented cultures lived in peace and harmony with equality between the sexes. The art, artifacts and earliest writings of these peoples documented that they were peaceful agriculturists, living harmoniously in matrilineal partnership societies.

The Feminine is Forgotten

All this began to change about five thousand years ago when warring tribes from northern Europe and central Asia descended into western Europe, the Near East and India. They invaded, conquered and destroyed the indigenous Goddess cultures.

It was a violent time when the patriarchal solar Gods overthrew the Mother Goddess. Women were stripped of their positions of political authority and their decision making powers as leaders. They were deprived of their spiritual authority as priestesses. Banned from functioning in their professional and healing capacities, they were progressively dis-empowered from expressing their sexuality, intelligence and self-sufficiency.

The emergence of the major world religions usurped the power of the feminine declaring that which once was sacred to be taboo. The Inquisition and witch hunts of the Middle

Ages was a determined effort by the Church and State to eliminate the last vestiges of the influence and power of the Goddess. It is estimated that, as many as, nine million women were systematically murdered during a three hundred year period.

The Patriarchy now ruled supreme. Inherent in this culture was blind obedience to the male principle, embodied by the father. It was based on the supremacy of the intellect, rigid rules, violence, control over others and the environment, efficiency and suppression of spontaneity and emotions. Women were relegated to second class citizens and considered the property of men. Women and all womanly functions were denigrated, defiled and became synonymous with evil.

Western civilization, embodying the legacy of patriarchy, has exalted all things male. It demands that women ignore or turn away from their hopes and dreams in deference to men and the demands of their families. The systematic stifling of the need for self-expression and self-actualization causes women enormous emotional pain. To stay out of touch with that pain, women have commonly used addictive substances and developed dysfunctional behaviors that have resulted in an endless cycle of abuse towards themselves, their bodies and others.

The five thousand year old patriarchal system is encoded within the very psyche of women. It has been passed down from generation to generation of women. It shapes their behaviors, attitudes and the very health of their bodies. It is the force that drives women to exhaustion, unable to stop long enough to attend to their own needs. It creates their obsession with a body that is never perfect enough. It is why women seek external authority to tell them how to live their own lives. It ensures that women remain economically, politically and spiritually helpless and dependent.

It is also the reason why women are filled with shame, disgust and guilt towards their bodies and normal female functions. It taunts them by calling menstruation 'the curse'. It is behind the millions of women who suffer each month with PMS—a symptom of their rejection of their feminine self.

It contributes to almost 50 percent of western women who have hysterectomies. It is why 60 percent of women experience painful periods each month—the majority of whom suffer in silence.

The Awakening

The re-emergence of the Feminine now stirring within the hearts of women is the call to reclaim all that has been kept hidden from them. Reclaiming this wisdom begins with honoring the cyclic nature of women. Women are lunar in nature. Just as the moon continues to cycle through its changes each month, so, too, do women. The menstrual cycle is the most basic, earthy cycle women have. The flow of blood is a woman's connection to the archetypal feminine. In many cultures, the menstrual cycle was viewed as sacred because it reconnects a woman with the creative principles of the universe.

The menstrual cycle governs not only the flow of fluids, but also information and creativity. The ebb and flow of dreams, intuition and hormones associated with different parts of the cycle offer women a profound opportunity to deepen their connection to their inner knowing.

Information is received and processed differently during each phase of the cycle. Brooke Medicine Eagle, Native American teacher and author affirms, "there is a spiritual power and beauty that builds in a woman who honors that part of herself. That's how women in native cultures got to be so wise."

Each month a woman recapitulates the phases of creation, nourishment, death and regeneration. From the first day of menstruation until ovulation is the follicular phase. During this time, her power can be used to conceive artistic and intellectual offspring as well as actual biological children.

It is the time when women are most outgoing and attractive to men (volatile hormones are secreted) and it culminates at the time of the full moon.

If pregnancy does not occur, the second half of the cycle is known as the luteal phase—from ovulation until the onset of menstruation. This is the time when there is a desire to retreat from outer activity to a more reflective mode. This inner space nurtures the opportunity to develop or give birth to something that comes from deep within. Menstruation correlates to the dark phase of the moon.

At this time women are most in tune with their inner knowing and understanding of what isn't working in their lives. Premenstrually, the 'veil between the worlds' of the seen and unseen, the conscious and the unconscious, is much thinner. It is when intuitive wisdom is the strongest and dreams most revealing. There is access to parts of the often unconscious self that are less available at all other times of the month. At this time women are able to connect to their magic—their ability to change things for the better because they are most sensitive to their inner selves.

In the Native American tradition, menstruating women would retire together to the moon lodge. This was a time for renewal and visioning. The women emerged afterward inspired and inspiring to others. Perhaps the majority of PMS cases would disappear if every modern woman gave herself permission to retreat from her duties for three or four days each month to her own personal 'moon lodge'.

Lunar Consciousness

The masculine world is based upon solar consciousness— the linear, rational, predictable rhythm of life. Lunar consciousness, however, requires listening and responding to the ever-changing inner impulses of instinctual wisdom. If a woman does not understand the need for slowing down and honoring the more introspective energy during the luteal phase, then intuitive information is unable to be received. This ignored information may then manifest as PMS or menopausal madness, in the same way that ignored feelings and bodily symptoms often result in disease. To the extent that women are out of touch with the hidden parts of themselves, they will suffer premenstrually and menopausally.

If a woman is in attunement with her menstrual wisdom, then each month she will be renewed and cleansed—physically, emotionally and spiritually. It was not necessary for Native American women to participate in the sweat lodge ceremony—a male ritual for purification—because it was understood that she was purified each month. Honoring such natural cycles can transform Premenstrual Syndrome into Premenstrual Strength.

The Truth About Menopause

If a woman is in harmony with her physical self as well as her deeper emotional and spiritual self, she is then prepared to enter the final initiation of her sacred woman's power—menopause.

In the patriarchal system, menopause has been made into the most dreaded and terrifying inevitability. Unlike men, who gain esteem and power as they age, menopausal women are perceived as losing their attractiveness and sexuality—literally and figuratively 'drying up'. How truly threatening this time is to women if their entire sense of worth is connected with being attractive to men. Menopause is also associated with loss of health, memory, independence, usefulness and creativity. In fact, most of the symptoms attributed to menopause are really the result of a stressful life-style which has created a huge imbalance in a woman's life and body.

The ancient Goddess cultures and many of today's indigenous cultures, knew the truth about menopause. It was the fullest blossoming of a woman's power, wisdom and creativity. Menopause was the initiation into the Wise Woman stage of life. In Native American tradition, it was only upon entering menopause that women were ready to become the Medicine Women and Shamans of their tribes. It was a position of the utmost respect.

For women to fulfil their potential during this second half of their lives, many myths must be shed. The conventional medical mind-set is that menopause is a deficiency disease not a natural process. It is believed to be a time when the ovaries dry up. Just as women's bodies have become pathologized and medicalized by the patriarchal, addictive system, so too has every function unique to women, menopause included.

As we have already explored, the ovaries go through changes during menopause, reducing estrogen and progesterone levels and altering their functions to produce other hormones. By no means do they shrivel up and cease functioning, as popular belief has it! In addition, other body sites such as the adrenal glands, skin, muscle, brain, pineal gland, hair follicles and body fat, are capable of making these essential hormones. Nature assists the female body to make healthy adjustments, in hormonal balance after menopause, providing a woman has taken good care of herself during the perimenopausal years.

In a most enlightening book called *Creative Menopause*, Farida Sharan states, "Menopause is a movement upwards. When we come into our forties and fifties, the tide of procreative sexuality and outward energies begins to shift inward and upward. As our ovaries release our last eggs and our hormones change, the challenge and the opportunity to open our higher centers of consciousness becomes a reality we face every day, either consciously or unconsciously. If we cling to what is already passing away, we get stuck. Disease patterns and mental and emotional imbalances are out of our refusal to move and change. But if we cooperate consciously with the process, the treasures that lie ahead will be greater than exploring the new world or space frontiers. Our unborn, uncharted being awaits to prepare us for our next level of emergence in the life of spirit."

She goes on to say, "When we complete menopause we move beyond the alternating cyclic nature and become like a direct current, charged and focused with the ability to speak and act truth and to express directly who we are through our inner vision. Certainly there is a tremendous shift of energy which is both liberating and powerful. We need to cooperate fully with this process to make the most of this creative opportunity. As attention shifts to the inner world, away from the personal into the universal, we learn to enjoy what is being given in our elder years and we do not want to waste time in fear and negativity by longing for what has already passed away."

Menopausal women have the opportunity to enter into a time of life fully empowered in their wisdom and creativity. It is the beginning of a whole new cycle of freedom and inner knowing.

The feminine path to power requires a woman to reclaim her own authority over her life—her needs, her rhythms and her body—and to trust her own instinctual nature once again. It's about realizing that she is not separate from nature but rather an expression of nature. Physical or emotional problems are expressions of disharmony. They are the messengers that let her know she is out of balance with some aspect of her life.

Self-healing requires personal disarmament, refusing to be at war any longer with a part of your body that's trying to tell you something. As women awaken, they will no longer need to deny or violate themselves in any way.

Shedding all the internalized messages of blame, self-doubt and self-hatred that are encoded within the cells frees each woman to attune to her inner guidance. Then she will always know when to be active and when to be quiet; when to care for others and when to care for self; when she is following her instinctual wisdom and when she is being directed by old conditioning. Therein lies her true source of power.

Like emerging from a long, deep period of hibernation, women all over the world are awakening to a power within themselves that has laid dormant for so very long. Feminine power is not the same as male power.

Feminine power emanates directly from a woman's wholeness. Only by reclaiming the banished sacred Feminine Self can women truly realize their deepest hopes and dreams for themselves, their families and Mother Earth.

Creating Sacred Feminine Power

The following are suggestions to support the blossoming of Women's Wisdom.

1. Journal—keep a daily account of your inner most thoughts and feelings.

2. Become aware of the moon and all her phases. Bask in the moonlight. Honor the moon as the archetype of the feminine. It has been shown that the light of the full moon increases levels of follicle stimulating hormone (FSH) via the hypothalamus and pituitary glands.

3. Take time either by yourself or with friends to have a full moon meditation.

4. Listen to your Menstrual Wisdom. When entering into the luteal stage, listen to your body. Take quiet time for yourself. Rest if you feel tired. Be daring and take a nap during the day! Allow your feelings to be expressed.

5. Keep a dream book to record your dreams and inner visions. Be especially aware of your dreams right before your period.

6. Buy a moon calendar to keep track of the moon's cycles each month.

7. Write into your diary when you will be experiencing your menstrual cycles.

8. Spend time alone with nature. Become aware of her rhythms and cycles, recognizing that you share her rhythms.

Recommended Reading:

Sister Moon Lodge: The Power and Mystery of Menstruation, Kisma Stepanich, Llewellyn Publications

Nostradamus: Prophecies for Women, Manuela Dunn Mascetti and Peter Lorie, Bloomsbury Publishing

Shakti Woman, Vicki Noble, Harper Collins Publishers

A Woman's Worth, Marianne Williamson, Random House

The Women's History of the World, Rosalind Miles, Paladin

Creative Menopause, Farida Sharan, Wisdome Press

Chapter 3

Women's Power and Women's Health Choices

The challenge of the modern woman is to be able to face the dragons of modern medicine, fully empowered, intuitive instincts intact and with the ability to say "No" if necessary. She also needs adequate self-esteem to set limits, to ask for what she wants and needs and the courage to seek and find all the appropriate guidance and support for her health needs.

The origins of disease are many—heredity, constitutional weaknesses, aging factors, life-style along with spiritual, mental and emotional causes. Even though there are times when we don't know why our body is giving us problems, we need to be open to exploring the ways that we have contributed to this "dis-ease" within ourselves. Have we been worrying excessively, not eating properly, or perhaps pushing ourselves to expend energy we don't have?

Whenever some illness is occurring, we must take some time and listen for the inner messages to discover what our body is trying to tell us. Instead of expecting doctors to be solely responsible for fixing us up, we need to learn to participate equally in our own healing process. While we can certainly appreciate modern medical skills and give thanks that they are available should we ever need them, we must not become a passive bystander regarding the needs of our own body. It is imperative that we become directly and therapeutically involved in our healing process—after all, who's body is it, anyway?

We can also learn how to adjust our daily lives, eliminating any habit that does not support our total well-being. We are now being asked to take a higher level of responsibility for our own lives.

Modern medicine developed out of mechanistic and scientific thinking that did not consider the important effects of the mind, emotions and spirit on our physical condition. This system disregards the whole person and focuses entirely on the physical. Modern medicine also regards the body as a machine and believes that when a part of the machine fails, the efficient treatment is to fix the part or replace it. True healing, which takes into account all aspects of a person's life, is rarely offered.

Orthodox medicine, based on this patriarchal, scientific paradigm, does not respect anything that cannot be logically and rationally seen, measured or proven. Much of life and death is invisible and immeasurable, as are feelings, thoughts and spiritual realities. The definable, measurable realities are only a small part of our life experience.

A New Understanding of the Mind/Body

Dr. Deepak Chopra, a pioneer of Mind/Body Medicine and author of the best selling book *Quantum Healing*, has said that our bodies are more like a flowing river rather than a sculpture frozen in time. Every thought, every emotion, every perception is directly and instantaneously affecting our bodies— either in the direction of healing or in the direction of disease.

We need to respect doctors and surgeons for their devoted years of study, their sacrifices and their remarkable skills. While this respect should not be eroded, neither should we regard them as the source of absolute control and authority over our bodies and our lives. We have the right to question or even refuse their suggestions for treatment. We must be fully informed and responsible for the decisions we make, the medicines we accept and whatever else we allow to be done to us. We do not have to offer ourselves up helplessly to the dictates of modern medicine.

We can co-operate fully and intelligently with the best of whatever is being offered medically and freely choose to explore other educational, therapeutic, natural, spiritual and complementary healing options.

The medical system is there to serve us. When we interact with doctors and the medical system, we must also be willing to challenge them to expand and grow. We must demand communication and respect. We must educate ourselves not only about our bodies but also the many psychological and spiritual changes that occur during a woman's life. As we discover the courage to seek out those who can help us, we must overcome feelings of fear, helplessness and despair. Whatever needs are not being provided for outside ourselves, we must now turn within, discovering the abundant strength and wisdom of our own inner resources.

When a menopausal woman seeks advice from her doctor for her health problems, the physical aspect of the menopausal symptoms usually becomes the focus. Menopause is often inaccurately blamed for other life-style, aging and disease symptoms. Generally a doctor is ill-equipped to understand and assist her with the spiritual unfolding and emotional transformation that is taking place. Everything is blamed on her hormones and the menopause. She is told that her ovaries are failing and the womb is often seen as irrelevant.

But menopause is not just a physical change, it is one of the most important spiritual stages in our life—an initiation into the blossoming of our Woman's Wisdom. Unfortunately, most women arrive at the time of menopause exhausted—physically, emotionally and mentally—from the relationship, family and work responsibilities that have consumed their attention for so many years of their lives. Since mid-life is a time of harvest, problems and issues that in the past have been ignored now surface demanding resolution. Life is demanding that we become the priority of our lives. Somehow we must find the time and energy to give to ourselves as we move through this passage. However much we have given of ourselves—to our loved ones, our work and our world—now is the time to fully give to ourselves. Such is the path to a woman's true power.

Women travel through many stages and initiations in their lives—from the onset of menstruation into motherhood and then menopause. With each stage, we must learn to make the necessary changes and adjustments that correspond to that time of life—with diet and life-style, emotional and creative expression and spiritual needs. Each stage is important and bestows upon us special gifts as we garner our learnings and wisdom throughout life.

Certainly women have it well within their own power not only to find safe, natural and effective ways to balance and heal themselves but to live long, full lives while preserving their vitality, youthfulness and health. Women deserve the right to appreciate themselves and their bodies through all the stages of life. As women find the way to return to a greater balance within themselves, they will profoundly know the truth of their immense contribution to Life.

Part Four —

Returning to Balance

Chapter 1

Walking the Middle Path

Buddha's greatest advice to the seekers of enlightenment was to walk the Middle Path. The Middle Path is about living in harmony and balance within ourselves. Finding balance is like walking a tight rope—each step along the wire requires rebalancing. Balance is a dynamic process; it changes with the days, the seasons, the years. To be so sensitive to oneself and one's needs that adjustments are made easily and quickly seems to be the key to living happily and peacefully. Welcoming change is an essential ingredient of the Middle Path. Without the willingness to change, the tight rope walker would quickly plunge to the ground.

Living life so that we may savor the many experiences along the way is an art. Life reveals its many secrets and wisdoms as we live it. The guides along this journey are our intuition, natural instincts and inner wisdom. They are the true jewels that we all possess. What is truly precious, however, may take a lifetime to discover.

To attain peace of mind it is essential to be committed to living in balance with oneself. Illness, emotional pain, unhappiness and confusion are merely symptoms of disharmony—they are the 'taps on our shoulders' attempting to tell us that we are out of sync with our Self in some way.

Restoring hormonal balance for a woman requires her to bring all aspects of her life into greater harmony and alignment. It is not just about taking some medication or treatment, no matter how natural. In every moment a woman's body is expressing her innermost needs. How adept she is at responding will reflect in her overall physical, emotional and mental well-being. There are times when we may fool ourselves. There are times when we can fool others. But we can never fool our body. It is the most sensitive barometer of our inner world.

A healthy plant has many requirements—the right amount of sun, correct temperature, adequate water, proper nutrients and careful weeding. All these factors are equally necessary for the plant's growth. We, too, have many requirements to sustain our growth. Balance is effortlessly attained if we honor and implement our essential ingredients for growth.

The following are suggestions for returning to balance. Some are absolutely essential while others fall into the category of optional choices. There are many ways to rebalance and each woman must find the way that is most appropriate and useful to her. Listen to your inner wisdom to find your way and have the courage to follow it.

Chapter 2

Food is Medicine

Proper understanding of diet is essential not only to a maintain a healthy body, but also for balanced emotions and an alert mind. The average western diet is hopelessly inadequate, out-of-balance and toxic.

Food is medicine for our body. Whatever we eat is either adding to our health or detracting from it. There is no middle ground. Learning the basic guidelines for eating is an obvious and necessary step for regaining balance.

Many excellent books abound that teach nutrition, so I will leave that to them. The following are some fundamental guidelines about what foods to include more often in your diet and what foods are best to reduce or avoid altogether. Scientific studies show that a mostly vegetarian, low-fat, wholefood diet is preventative medicine at its finest. Eating organic food— vegetables, fruits, seeds, grains and meats— is becoming a necessity due to mounting evidence of the long-term harm herbicides, pesticides and other xeno-estrogens are doing to our health.

There is some new information about what foods are good for women, so that will be the focus in this section. Lissa De Angelis and Molly Siple, two nutritional counsellors, have co-authored an excellent cookbook book called *Recipes for Change* to assist women to return to hormonal balance through food.

I have included their most up-to-date findings which include new nutritional stars such as bioflavonoids, boron, phytohormones and essential fatty acids.

These nutrients, which are found in countless foods, play numerous roles in supporting a woman's body during its many changes.

Bioflavonoids

This group of compounds (which includes citron, hesperidin, rutin and flavanones) has a structure and chemical activity similar to estrogen. By mimicking and modulating estrogen fluctuations, the presence of bioflavonoids in the body has been shown to control hot flashes and the psychological symptoms of menopause including anxiety, irritability and mood swings. Bioflavonoids lessen heavy menstrual bleeding in premenopause, strengthen capillary walls and help to keep the skin healthy and supple. Some of the foods that contain bioflavonoids include green peppers, cherries, buckwheat, rose hips and, especially, citrus, which contains the complete bioflavonoid complex. Bioflavonoids are not destroyed by cooking but remain stable.

Boron

Throughout your life sufficient boron is needed for metabolizing calcium as well as for maintaining motor skills and mental alertness. Two large apples, a cup of broccoli florets or a handful of nuts supplies 1 mg. of boron, a good start for the 1 to 3 mgs of boron per day required for good health.

Some other boron-containing foods include millet, buckwheat, whole oats and barley, soybeans, lentils, spinach, potatoes, parsley, beets, green peas, cabbage, asparagus, pears, peaches, grapes, raisins, rockmelons, lemons, bananas, almonds, hazelnuts, walnuts, flax seeds and shrimp. Interestingly, a recent study of women on estrogen replacement therapy seems to indicate that boron can mimic and enhance the action of supplemental estrogen.

Phytohormones

Sometimes called phytoestrogens, phytohormones are substances found in plant foods that affect your hormone status. They are present in dozens of foods that we commonly eat and these foods have been shown to have an effect on the hormonal balance of the body. Phytohormone potencies are considerably weaker than the estrogen that is produced in your ovaries, called estradiol. Although many of these plant hormones are 1/400th to 1/100,000th the potency of estradiol, they can mimic and modulate estrogens and can help stabilize hormone fluctuations. Some of the phytohormone foods are brown rice, beans, flax seeds, radishes, tofu, pomegranates, rhubarb, potatoes, fennel and green tea. Vegetarian women can have phytohormone levels one hundred times greater than women eating a typical western diet.

Consuming foods rich in phytohormones may also lower your risk of heart disease and breast cancer. Japanese women eating a traditional diet have fewer incidences of hot flashes and lower rates of breast cancer. Scientists have suggested that the consumption of soybeans and soy products like tofu, which are high in phytohormones, is part of the reason.

However, the traditional Japanese diet is also low in processed and refined foods and high in mineral-rich seaweed and fresh fish oils—all of which are important factors. It is interesting to note that when Japanese women eat a more western diet, the incidence of heart disease and cancer increases.

Essential Fatty Acids

Essential fatty acids make up the components of many organs and tissues. They bring oxygen to our tissues, help prevent premenstrual symptoms, improve the condition of hair, nails and skin and help prevent all major degenerative diseases, including heart disease and cancer. They are essential for good health throughout life.

There are two families of essential fatty acids, called omega-6 and omega-3. We need about twice as much omega-6 as omega-3. However, most of us are already getting so much omega-6 that we need to seriously boost our consumption of omega-3. Some of the foods high in omega-3 are walnuts, flax seed oil, dark green leafy vegetables and fish. The average healthy adult requires 4 teaspoons of essential oils per day, but a woman in menopause, especially with dry skin, hair and vaginal tissue, may need to 2 or 3 tablespoons per day before her symptoms disappear.

Chapter 3

Foods to Avoid

Refined Sugar

Refined sugars (cane and beet sugar, brown sugar, corn syrup and any word that ends in 'ose', ie dextrose) are completely devoid of vitamins, minerals and fibre and have no nutritive value. They stress your body and actually deplete it of vitamins and minerals. Refined sugar can lead to calcium loss and contributes to weight gain, diabetes, tooth and gum disorders, nervous disorders, low blood sugar and fatigue.

Caffeine

Caffeine quickens respiration, increases blood pressure, stimulates the kidneys, excites brain function and temporarily alleviates fatigue and depression. It can create vitamin and mineral deficiencies, prevent iron absorption, irritate the stomach lining, aggravate the heart and arteries and increase nervous symptoms. Caffeine is found in coffee, black teas, chocolate and in many sodas. Coffee is a diuretic. It has few nutrients and stimulates excess excretion of urine along with the vitamins and minerals urine contains.

Processed Oils

Most cooking oils are refined which means that they have had the flavorful elements, smells and natural colors removed. Corn, canola and safflower oils are all refined. Refined oils contain toxic substances and should be avoided. Hydrogenated fats, such as shortening and margarine, are strongly linked to heart disease and cancer. The beneficial oils are extra-virgin olive oil, flax seed oil, unrefined sesame oil and unsalted butter. Ideally, oils should be organically produced and cold-pressed. Always keep oils refrigerated or they will go rancid.

Refined Flours and Grains

The most nutritional part of the grain (the germ and bran) is removed when processed, leaving the part we buy highly devoid of vitamins, minerals, fibre and essential fatty acids. All whole grains are correctly called complex carbohydrates consisting of the bran, germ and endosperm. Whole grains include whole wheat, brown rice, buckwheat, millet, cornmeal, oatmeal and whole grain pastas. Whenever possible choose products made with whole grains.

Dairy Products

Dairy products are best avoided completely. Contrary to all the dairy industry advertising, it is one of the worst foods a woman can eat. Consumption of dairy products increases symptoms of PMS such as swelling, cramping and breast tenderness.

After abstaining from all dairy products (a moderate amount of unsalted butter is acceptable since it is primarily a fat containing very little milk solids or protein) many women have reported shrinking or disappearance of fibroids, less menstrual bleeding and for fewer days, reduced endometriosis pain, improved allergies and sinusitis and lessening of recurrent vaginitis.

Dairy products also contain many added hormones and residues of antibiotics. Dairy foods are a protein. Excessive protein leaches calcium from the bone in order to neutralize the more acidic environment that the proteins create. Therefore dairy products contribute to bone loss!

It is no coincidence that the countries with the highest rates of osteoporosis—the United States, Great Britain and Sweden—are also the countries with the highest dairy consumption.

A Word About Vitamins

It is currently estimated that less than 9 percent of the population eats an adequate amount of vegetables and fruits to maintain high levels of vitamins and minerals in our bodies. Many women throughout their lives are missing vital nutrients. No wonder ill health is so common. While vitamin and mineral tablets are a useful way of supplementing nutrients, they must be taken in conjunction with nutrient-rich food. Together with these foods, supplements can build and fuel a depleted body. Taking supplements without accompanying food is like giving water to a flowerpot that has no plant. Be sure to get proper nutritional advice when choosing vitamins. Just remember, popping vitamin pills will never replace wholesome nutrition.

Recommended Reading:

Recipes for Change, Lissa De Angelis and Molly Siple, Penguin Books

Menopause Without Medicine, Linda Ojeda, Ph.D., Hunter House, Inc. Publishers, California

Lick the Sugar Habit, Nancy Appleton, Ph.D., Paragon Press, Pennsylvania

Chapter 4

Precious Water

When it comes to rebalancing the body, one of the most crucial ingredients is generally overlooked— and that is the most precious, life-giving element on this planet, water! Did you know that water is necessary for optimum brain function, digestion, absorption of nutrients, circulation, hormonal management and all biochemical processes in each of your cells? It is excellent for healthy, clear, soft skin. Scientific research has shown that the better the water management in a cell, the more efficiently proteins, enzymes, hormones and other biochemical elements are able to function. Dehydration can create an imbalance of minerals which will disrupt hormone balance.

So important is the need for proper hydration that the newsletter, *Health Alert*, reported recently, "When it comes to disease like heart, kidney or stomach disease, allergies, asthma, arthritis and skin disease, your state of hydration (water balance) may be the single most important factor in your recovery or even your survival".

Of particular and critical interest to women is the role of chronic dehydration in the development of breast cancer. In his book, *Your Body's Many Cries for Water*, Dr. Batmanchelidj says that the stress that dehydration creates "will increase the secretion of a hormone called prolactin which can at times cause the breast to transform into cancerous tissue. Also, the dehydration would alter the balance of amino acids and allow more DNA errors during cell division."

Dr. Batmanchelidj goes on to say that, "The breast is a water-secreting organ...Whether you are having a child or not makes no difference. The breast must be ready to fulfill its predestined role...If a woman already has breast cancer, drinking plenty of water would assist with any therapy by flushing out the toxins. If you do not have breast cancer or want to prevent a metastasis from occurring, it is urgent that you drink enough water. If you don't, your breast may suffer horribly because of its unique role in supplying fluids."

A serious problem these days is a chronic state of dehydration in women. When thirsty it is common to drink coffee, tea, fruit juices, sodas and energy drinks. Unfortunately these drinks do not hydrate the body but rather contribute to dehydration. Only pure water will do! Tap water is generally so polluted with chemical concoctions that it is also dehydrating. Either filtered water or bottled water is the better choice. Generally a woman needs about 1-1.5 liters per day—whether she is thirsty or not!

Hydration is the body's ability to absorb and manage water effectively. Hydration is one of the keys to more energy and improved immunity. It is not how much water you drink but rather how well hydrated your body is. The stresses of daily living—pollution, emotional and physical stress, or inadequate nutrition—can all compromise your body's water balancing mechanism. Simply drinking more water is not always the answer. Just as when water is poured onto a really dried up potted plant and most of it runs right out the bottom, even though you may be drinking lots of water, it too may be pouring right out of you without hydrating your body. The key is getting the body to absorb the water efficiently.

A great way to improve hydration is to drink water regularly throughout the day, especially if you can drink several glasses made with 20 percent apple juice. The sugar of the diluted apple juice enhances hydration.

Recommended Reading:

1. *The Water You Drink* by John Archer, Pure Water Press, NSW, Australia

2. *Your Body's Many Cries for Water*, Dr. F. Batmanchelidj, Global Health Solutions

Chapter 5

The Breath of Life

Breathing, like proper water intake, is so often overlooked in our quest for greater balance in our lives. Yet proper breathing is a vital key for assisting longevity, creating balanced hormonal production, increasing energy and reducing stress. It also optimizes athletic performance, enhances concentration and increases confidence. Proper breathing returns our body to balance—physically, emotionally, mentally and spiritually. Filling our body with oxygen is filling it with Life Force. No wonder that breathing has been an intrinsic part of all the ancient wisdoms throughout history.

The key to receiving the healing benefits from the breath is to breathe properly—the way we were designed to breathe. While most people tend to breathe rapidly and only in their upper chest while raising their shoulders as they inhale deeply this, in fact, is known as futile breathing. It is a disastrous breathing style!

Dr. Saul Hendler, a respected medical doctor, comments in his book, *The Oxygen Breakthrough—30 Days to an Illness-free Life*, that futile breathing can cause cardiac symptoms, angina, respiratory symptoms, gastro-intestinal distress, anxiety, panic, depression, headache, dizziness, seizures, increased susceptibility to infection and other immune dysfunctions and sleep disturbances. In addition, futile breathing contributes to confused thinking and emotional upset.

A recent article published in the *American Journal of Obstetrics and Gynecology* (167;436-7) reported that slow, deep breathing reduced the incidence of hot flashes by 50 per cent in a group of women who were not on hormone replacement therapy.

Receiving the optimum benefit from the breath, which is really the way nature designed us to breathe, requires drawing the inhaled air all the way down into the very bottom of the lungs so that the diaphragm expands. It's as though the breath were sinking all the way down and then gradually inflating the rest of the lungs. You have taken a correct breath when you are able to fill your lungs fully without lifting your shoulders! The inhale is the more active part of the breath and the exhale is very gentle and relaxed.

I teach this simple breathing technique in my psychotherapy practice with the most profound results. My clients experience feelings of profound peace, mental clarity, emotional balance, an expanded awareness, inner realizations, increased energy and relief from a wide variety of physical problems including hormonal imbalance. I recommend practicing the following breathing exercise for just twenty breaths, twice a day.

The Healing Breath

1. Sitting or lying comfortably, place your hands on your stomach (abdomen).

2. Inhale slowly and deeply through your nose, letting your abdomen expand as though you were filling up the bottom part of a balloon.

3. Allow the breath to first be drawn into the lower lungs, then gradually allow it to fill the upper lungs as well.

4. Relax and gently exhale.

5. Guide the breath into a circular rhythm so that the breath can flow easily from the inhale to the exhale without pausing or stopping.

6. As you feel greater relaxation in your body, allow the inhale to gently expand, taking in fuller breaths.

Chapter 6

Use It or Lose It

Nature designed the body to move. Exercise is an important and essential ingredient for physical and emotional health. It not only tones up your muscles but works on your whole anatomy. It works in conjunction with your metabolism for the better handling of nutrients. In fact, exercise added to nutrients upgrades their effectiveness and efficiency. According to one study, women of childbearing age who exercised four or more hours per week halved their risk of breast cancer before menopause.

Regular exercise will also decrease your risk of heart disease by raising the level of good HDL and lowering bad LDL. It is not surprising that sedentary women are three times more likely to die of heart attacks than women who exercise regularly. You can reduce your risk of dying from a heart attack by 50 percent if you tend to be at risk for heart disease. (By the way, this is the same figure that's been used for Premarin!) Exercise is also directly linked to your hormonal health which is why hot flashes can be reduced by a regular exercise program.

Exercise is beneficial at whatever age you begin. Dr. Deepak Chopra relates a study in his book *Ageless Body, Ageless Wisdom* conducted by gerontologists at Tufts University. They visited a nursing home where they selected a group of the most frail residents and put them on a weight-training regimen.

Within eight weeks wasted muscles had come back by 300 percent, coordination and balance improved and overall a sense of active life returned. What makes this accomplishment truly wondrous, however, is that the youngest subject in the group was 87 and the oldest 96!

The real trick to exercise is to like what you do. If the kind of exercise you're doing is more like duty or drudgery, then the benefits won't be as great if you found something that was thoroughly enjoyable. For me, rollerblading is an absolute delight. I can happily cruise along on my blades for hours at a time. The time I'm getting my aerobic exercise also fills me with a great sense of pleasure. So, choose your exercise with enjoyment in mind!

To strengthen your bones, some form of weight bearing exercise must be included in your program. Walking uphills, bicycling in low gear, weight training, climbing steps or doing a step machine are all examples providing bone strengthening benefits.

Researchers in St. Louis found that in less than 22 months women who exercised at least three times a week increased their bone density 5.2 percent while sedentary women actually lost 1.2 percent. A recently reported randomized controlled study from Canada found that subjects who exercised for 60 minutes three times a week for a year stabilized their bone mass, improved their cardiovascular endurance and had a better overall sense of well-being than those in the control group.

Recommended Reading:

Better Bones, Better Body, Susan E. Brown Ph.D.,
Keats Publishing, CT

Strong Women Stay Young, Marian E. Nelsen, Ph.D.,
Bantam Books, New York, NY

Chapter 7

Meditation—Moving Inwards

While meditation may conjure up images of exotic, esoteric techniques, it is in fact simply learning to settle one's thoughts and to be fully focused in the moment. It offers a time for inner contemplation. There are many ways to attain that centering. Some can be learned through various techniques taught at meditation/relaxation centers or from audio or video tapes. It is also possible to meditate as one listens to favorite music or while just strolling along the beach or in a park. Whatever your preferred way may be, taking time to meditate has clearly been shown to produce marvellous benefits both for one's physical health as well as emotional and spiritual well-being. Besides eliminating the harmful effects of stress, it enables you to tap into your creative energy and even reverse the aging process!

To receive meditation's many rewards, it is only necessary to set aside 15 - 20 minutes each day. A simple meditation technique involves finding a quiet time and then to simply follow your breath flowing in and out. As soon as you notice your mind wandering, gently bring it back to the breath. It's that easy! It is also important to remember that making this quiet time a priority in your life is really about valuing yourself.

For many years I was very erratic with my meditation practices. Since committing to daily meditation time (which for me is early in the morning) I have found more emotional balance.

Things just don't seem to cause the reactive responses in me that they once did. I guess you could call it a growing sense of inner peace. My morning meditation time is now a regular part of my life.

Chapter 8

Loving Your Body

A very special Hawaiian elder named Angeline Locey, the founder of a wonderful healing center on the island of Kauai, taught me about the importance of loving the body. She would always chant, "Malama Pono Ea Oi," as she lovingly massaged people's bodies. Translated it means, " I take back my body, I love my body." Over and over again, Angeline would remind everyone to love their bodies. She said that without the love for our bodies we can never be truly whole and healed.

Loving our body is certainly a challenge for most women. Our body seems to be our enemy. It's never quite perfect enough to please us. Somehow, the more we starve it, deny it and despise it, the more we add to our own self-hatred. How can it be otherwise? After all, we are our bodies. Learning to love and appreciate the uniqueness of our bodies, whatever the shape, characteristics or condition it may be in, is reclaiming the love for ourselves. And the secret is that the more we learn to love our bodies, the more they transform into the bodies we love!

There are many ways to begin loving your body. It can be as simple as indulging in sensuous bath, complete with candles, music and aromatherapy bath oil. It is certainly a wonderful opportunity to relax and dissolve muscle tensions.

An aromatherapy body rub is another loving gesture. It is best done after a shower or bath. Add a few drops of your favorite aromatherapy oil into a capful of massage oil. Then with your finger tips gently massage the oil all over your body, beginning with the soles of the feet and moving all the way up to your head. Since you are using just a small amount of oil, it is quickly absorbed. As you massage, send loving thoughts to your body.

Other gestures of love may include receiving regular massages, taking time out in nature, afternoon naps, getting cuddles and eating nutritious foods. Discover your favorite ways or explore new ones. One thing is for sure, without learning to love your body, true inner harmony will always elude you.

For more information about the healing retreats and services available at Angeline's healing center contact:

Angeline Locey
P.O. Box 567
Anahola, Kauai 96703
Hawaii USA

Tel:/Fax: (808) 822-3235

Chapter 9

Emotional Healing and Spiritual Growth

Healing emotional pain is one of the purposes of this life time. It is called growth. We are truly blessed to be living in a time when we no longer need to keep our inner pain hidden away—eating away at our self-love, joy and creativity. Personal growth is becoming more widely accepted as a legitimate need of all people. There are so many wonderful resources presently available to anyone who truly desires to free themselves of the hurt of the past in order to live a more fulfilling life. Through the myriad of counselling techniques, seminars, classes, support groups, body work modalities, alternative healing methods and personal awareness books, tapes and videos, we are given countless opportunities to explore ourselves and shed old, outmoded ways of perceiving reality.

As women raised in a culture that has favored masculine values such as competition, hierarchy, control, rational thinking, obedience to authority and violence, we carry many wounds within us. These are the wounds handed down to us from the many past generations of women who were made to be silent, to feel powerless, guilt-ridden and worthless. Such emotional wounds blind us to the true beauty, wisdom and love of who we are. Perhaps the wide-spread disharmony presently manifesting within women's bodies is merely a reflection of generations who lived in denial of their Selves.

In Grace Gawler's book, *Women of Silence: The Emotional Healing of Breast Cancer*, she explores the hidden side of cancer—the emotional aspect of illness. "Although there are visible lumps on and in the body, these symptoms may actually have their origins within the soul where the creative threads of life dwell. When there are blocks in the creative flow of a woman's life and when the expression of that creativity is blocked, her creative knots can become knotted into what are unhealthy 'knots of the soul'. These 'knots' are formed by frustrated emotional energy at a very deep level of the psyche.

"Interestingly, women dealing with breast cancer almost always have a history of unresolved emotional pain throughout their life." These are the shackles that must be released.

As though awakening from a long sleep, women all over the world are returning to honor the wise woman within. Emotional healing is the path which leads to greater spiritual awareness—the awareness of a reality where all life is bound together with invisible threads of love.

Recommended Reading:

Anatomy of The Spirit, Caroline Myss, Ph.D.,
Bantam Books

The Creation of Health, Norman Shealy, M.D., Ph.D. and Carolyn Myss, Stillpoint Publishing

Love, Medicine and Miracles, Bernie Siegel, M.D.,
Harper & Row Publishers

Women of Silence: The Emotional Healing of Breast Cancer,
by Grace Gawler, Hill of Content, Victoria Australia

Chapter 10

Coming Full Circle

Many thousands of years ago, forgotten by history but not by the memories in our bones, the feminine principle as embodied by women, gave rise to the flourishing of the cultures where nature and all of life was recognized. Women were honored as representatives of nature's beauty, wisdom and the mysteries of life. It was a time when women were so finely attuned to life's secrets that they were the spiritual and political leaders, the healers, the artisans and educators.

As the full moon wanes, so too do all things. Not as decline and death but rather as change and growth. As the light of those feminine cultures was eclipsed by the new male-dominated world, all that was once held sacred became profane. The gifts and strengths of women were turned into weaknesses and faults. Women were defiled and perceived as less than human—and treated accordingly. Women learned from men to hate themselves and their bodies. Their only value came from either child bearing and child rearing or as sources of men's sexual pleasure.

But we now move once again slowly towards the light. We are coming to the end of this dark moon phase of history. It is no coincidence that women are rejecting all the ways that have usurped their true power and true instinctual wisdom.

Regaining an appreciation of her body is an essential part of a woman's re-awakening. While the Pill appeared at a time of history when women demanded their sexual freedom and independence we now know, without a doubt, that the short-term benefits have demanded a terrible price. Filling our bodies with drugs that stopped our natural flow of hormones not only unbalanced our bodies they also disconnected us from our feminine cyclic wisdom—the very heart and soul of a woman.

It is becoming evident that the Pill no longer serves the empowerment of women. It sounds a death knell—if not the death of women's bodies, surely the death of their spirit. It is only by embracing the wisdom of nature, natural cycles, natural medicines, natural foods and natural rhythms that women will find their wholeness and themselves. Success-ful and healthy contraception and conception are a part of woman's initiation into her own mystery which she has denied herself for so long.

Menopause is another initiation into women's mysteries. It does not need to be successfully 'managed'. It is not a dis-ease condition that must be controlled or overcome. It does not, under normal conditions, necessitate drugs, surgery or manipulation of our bodies into unnatural processes. It is a rite of passage that all women must make. The need is for menopause to be a time for women to be honored, nurtured, understood and celebrated.

Real healing can only be attained by returning to inner balance, perhaps for the very first time in one's life. For thousands of years, the vast majority of women throughout the planet have lived their lives without realizing just how disconnected they were from themselves. There is much that we, as women, have forgotten about our innate wisdom and healing nature. There is also much that we have been taught to disdain about ourselves and out bodies. Now it is time to remember! It's time for the tying together of all the threads that weave the magnificent tapestry of a woman's wholeness. Life is beckoning us to return to balance for the sake of ourselves, our future generations and our planet.

Sources forNatural Hormones and Other Natural Products

Bajamar Women's Healthcare Pharmacy
9609 Dielman Rock island
St. Louis, MO 63132
(800) 255- 8025
(transdermal natural progesterone an other natural hormone products)

Madison Pharmacy Associates
429 Gammon Pl.
Madison , WI 53719
(800) 558 704
(transdermal natural progesterone an other natural hormone products)

Pacific Research Laboratories
1010 Crenshaw Blvd., Suite 170
Torrance, CA 90275
(310) 320-2232
(310) 320 7557 Fax
(Nutritional supplements, yam cream)

Sun Valley Herb Company
331 1st Avenue North
Ketchum, ID 83340
(208) 726-4790
(herbs, homeopathic, menopausal products)

Transitions for Health
621 S.W. Alder St., Suite 900
Portland, OR 97205
(800) 888 6814
(800) 944-0168 Fax
(Transdermal natural progesterone and other women's products)

Women's International Pharmacy
5708 Monona Dr.
Madison, WI 53716
(800) 279 5708
(transdermal natural progesterone an other natural hormone products)

Doctor Referral Listings and Support Organizations

American Association of Naturopathic Physicians
2366 East Lake Ave. East, Suite 322
 Seattle, WA
(206) 328-8510

Alliance for Alternatives in Healthcare,
P.O. Box 6279
 Thousand Oaks, CA 91359-6279
(805) 494-7818

Health World
Excellent on-line resource for complimentary medicine.
Provides free access to Medline
hhtp:// healthy.net

HERS (Hysterectomy Educational Resources and Services)
422 Bryn Mawr Ave.
Bala Cynwyd, Pennsylvania 19004
(610) 667-7757

International Academy of Compounding Pharmacists
With approximately 900 members in the United States,
Canada and Australia, they will assist in finding a com-
pounding pharmacist near you.
P.O. Box 1365
Sugarland, Texas 77487
(800) 927 4227
(713) 933-9215

National Center for Homeopathy
801 N. Fairfax St. , # 306
Alexandria, VA 22314
(705) 548-7790
(703) 548-7792 Fax

Natural Woman Institute (888-489-6629)
Outreach and education for women about plant-derived
hormones, how a woman's body works at mid-life, and how
important hormonal balance is to keeping her healthy, active
and vital. They provide an updated database of doctor
referrals.

North Eastern Herbal Association
PO Box 146
Marshall, VT 05658
(802) 456 1402

Newsletters

Dr. Julian Whitaker's *Health and Healing ,Newsletter*
Phillips Publishing , Inc.
7811 Montrose Road
Potomac, Maryland 20854
(800) 211 8561

Christian Northrup, M.D. *Health Wisdom for Women*
Phillips Publishing , Inc.
7811 Montrose Road
Potomac, Maryland 20854
(800) 211 8561

Menopause News
2074 Union Street
San Francisco, CA 94123
800-241-MENO
email: mnews@well.com

References:

Chapter 1

1. Germaine Greer, *The Change*, Hamish Hamilton, London, 1991
2. John Archer, *Bad Medicine* Simon & Schuster, Australia, 1995, p.217
3. Ibid., p. 192
4   Ibid., p. 211
5. Sandra Coney, *The Menopause Industry*, Spinnifex Press Pty Ltd., Australia, 1991, P. 164-165

Chapter 2

1. Betty Kamen Ph.D.

Chapter 3

1. Marshall, E. "Search For A Killer: Focus Shifts From Fats To Hormones", 1993, *Science* 259: 616-617
2. (a) Dumble, Lynette J., Ph.D., M.Sc., " Odds Against Women with Heart Disease", presented at Health Sharing Women's Forum, Royal College of Surgeons, Melbourne, Victoria, Australia, 14 September, 1995.
    (b) Barrett-Connor, Elisabeth, "Heart Disease in Women", *Fertility and Sterility* (1994), 62(2):1275-132S.

Chapter 4

1. *Menopause News*, Vol. Issue 2 March/April p2
2. *Health Action*, November/December 1985
3. Ibid.

Chapter 5

1. John R. Lee, MD, *What Your Doctor May Not Tell You About Menopause*, Warner Books, New York, 1996 p. 67-68
2. John R. Lee, MD, *Natural Progesterone: The Multiple Role of a Remarkable Hormone*, BLL Publishing, California, 1993, p. 8
3. Ibid., p. 29
4. Lee, op.cit., p. 121
5. Ibid., p. 131
6. Ibid., p. 132

Chapter 6

1. Nancy Beckham, *"Why Women Should Not Take HRT"*, *WellBeing Magazine*, No. 67, p. 70
2. Ellen Brown and Lyn Walker, *"Menopause and Estrogen*, Frog Ltd., CA. 1996, p. 25
3. *Australian Doctor*, August 29, 1997, p. 3

Chapter 8

1. Nancy Beckham, *Menopause - A Positive Approach Using Natural Therapies*, Penguin Books Australia Lt. 1995 p. 36-37
2. Ibid., p. 36
3. *British Medial Bulletin*, 1992, 48:458-68

Chapter 9

1. *Newsweek*, March 18, 1996
2. Leslie Kenton, *Passage to Power*, Random House, London, 1995, p. 34
3. John Archer -*The Water You Drink, How Safe Is It?*, Pure Water Press, 1996, p. 34

Chapter 9 (cont)

4.   Leslie Kenton, op. cit., p. 32
5.   Diane Clorfene-Casten, *"Breast Cancer, Poisons, Profits and Prevention"*, Common Courage Press, Maine, 1996, p. 33-34
6.   John R. Lee, MD *What Your Doctor May Not Tell You About Menopause*, p. 51
7.   Ibid., p. 56
8.   *Wheel of Hormones*, Lars Mortensen, TV2 Denmark, T.V. Production, 1995
9.   *Green Left Weekly*, June 19, 1996

Chapter 10

1.   Lee, op. cit., p. 44
2.   *Menopause News*, Vol. Issue 2 March/April p. 2
3.   Lee, Jane Lue, "Biomarkers and Prevention", *Cancer Epidemiology*, 1996, 3:65-70

Chapter 11

1.   Lee, op. cit., p. 325
       Menopause, Warner Books, New York, 1996 p. 325
2.   *Menopause News*, Vol. Issue 2 March/April p. 1

Chapter 12

1.   Kate Neil. *Balancing Hormones Naturally*, ION Press, London, 1994. p. 28
2.   John Wilks, *A Consumers Guide To The Pill*, TGB Book, Australia, 1996, p. 81
3.   Ibid, pp. 59-60
4.   Kate Neil, *Balancing Hormones Naturally*, ION Press, London, 1994. p. 28

Chapter 13

1.   *Partners, The AIM News Magazine*, August 1996, p. 22

Chapter 14

1.   Lee, op. cit., p. 258
2.   Racquel Martin, *The Estrogen Alternative*, Healing Arts Press, Vermont, 1997. p. 109
3.   Lee, op. cit. p. 42
4.   Christiane Northrup, MD, *Women's Bodies, Women's Wisdom*, Bantam Books, New York p. 158
5.   John R. Lee, MD., *Natural Progesterone*, p. 87
6.   John R. Lee, MD., op. cit. p. 254
7.   Ibid. p. 259
8.   Ibid. p. 244
9.   John R. Lee, *MD., What Your Doctor May Not Tell You About Menopause*, p. 103
10   Martin, op. cit., p. 43
11. Ibid. p. 230
12. Martin, op. cit., p. 52
13. Lee, op. cit., p. 147
14. Ibid. p. 238
15. Brown and Walker, op. cit., p. 93

Chapter 16

1.   Marcus Laux, ND., and Christine Conrad, *Natural Woman, Natural Menopause*, Harper Collins, New York, 1997, p. 79
2.   Henry M. Leman, et al, "Reduced Estriol Excretun In Patients With Breast Cancer Prior To Endocrine Therapy", *Journal Of American Medical Association*, 196 (1966): p. 1128-34

Chapter 16 (cont)

3.   Alvin Follingstad, "Estriol For The Forgotten Estrogen", *Journal of American Medical Association*, 239, No.1 (January 2, 1978): p. 29-30

4.   Walter E. Stamm and Raul Raz, "A Controlled Trial Of Intravaginal Estriol In Post Menopausal Women With Recurrent Urinary Tract Infections", *Journal Of American Medical Association*, 329, No. 11 (September 9 1993) p. 753-56

Chapter 17

1.   D. T. Felson, et al, "The Effect Of Post Menopausal Estrogen Therapy On Bone Density In Elderly Women", *New England Journal Of Medicine*, 329 (1993): pp. 1141-462

2.   C. Christinssen, et al, "Bone Mass In Post Menopausal Women After The Withdrawal Of Estrogen/Progesterone Therapy", *Lancet*, February 29, 1982: p. 459-61

3.   Neil, op. cit., p. 46

4.   Kenton, op. cit., p. 19-20

5.   Ibid p. 19-20

6.   Lee, J. R., Osteoporosis Reversal: the Role of Progesterone. Intern. Clin. Nutr. Rev. 1990, 10:384-391

7.   William Regelson, *The Super Hormone Promise*, Simon & Schuster, New York, 1996, p. 186

8.   Love, R. R., et. al., "Effects Of Tamoxifen On Women With Breast Cancer", *New England Journal Of Medicine*, 1992, 326: p. 853-6

9.   Welton, DC Kempa HCG Post GB Van Stavneren, "A Meta-Analysis Of The Effects For Calcium Intake On Bone Mass In Young, Middle-Aged Females And Males", 1995, WA Nutrition, 125:2802-2813

10.   Lee, op. cit., p. 183

11.   Love, op. cit., p.97

Chapter 17 (cont)

12. Lee, op. cit., p. 189
13. Myagawa, K., Rosch, J., Stanczk, F. and Hermesmeyer, K., "Medroxyprogesterone Interferes With Ovarian Steroid Protection Against Coronary Vasospasm", *Nature Medicine*, 1997, 3:273-274
14. Sullivan, J. M., shala Bashau, A., Miller, L. A., Lerner, J. L., and MacBrayer, J. D., "Progestin Enhances Vasoconstrictor Responses In Postmenopausal Women Receiving Estrogen Replacement." *Menopause Journal of North American Menopause Society*, 1995: 2 (4): 193-199
15. Nancy Beckham, op. cit., p. 42-43
16. Lee, op. cit., p. 197
17. Love, op. cit., p.113
18. *Austrialian Doctor*, "Breast Risk Double With Long Term HRT", August 29, 1997, p.1
19. Lee, op. cit., p. 208
20. King-Jen Chuang MD, Tigris T.Y. Lee, MD, Gustavo Linares-Cruz, MD, Sabine Fournier, Ph.D. Bruno de Ligneires, MD, "Influences Of Percutaneous Administration Of Estradiol And Progesterone On Human Breast Epithelial Cell Cycle In Vivo. *Fertility and Sterility* April 1995; 63:4 785-791
21. *Journal Of The National Cancer Institute*, 1996: vol 88, 643-49
22. Wilson, P.W.F., Garrison R J, Castelli W P, "Post Menopausal Estrogen Use, Cigarette Smoking And Cardiovascular Morbidity In Women Over 50", The Framingham Study, *New England Journal Of Medicine*, 1985; 313:17, 11038-43
23. Love, op. cit., p.264
24. Beckham, op. cit., p. 48
25. Neil, op. cit., p. 40
26. Clarfene - Casten, op. cit., p. 101
27. Northrup, op. cit., p. 471
28. Kenton op. cit., p. 94

29.   Lee, op. cit., p. 220

30.   Rodriguez, C., Calle, E. E., Coates, R. J., Miracle-McMahill, H. L., Thun, M. J., and Heath, C. W. Jr., "Estrogen Replacement Therapy And Fatal Ovarian Cancer." *American Journal Of Epidemiology 1995; 141(9) : 828-835*

31.   Ellerbrook, J.M., Lee, J.A.H. "Oral contraceptives and malignant melanoma", *Journal of the American Medical Association* 1968;206:649

32.   *The Walnut Creek Contraceptive Drug Study* Vol III, NIH Pub. 1986 and including Beral,V., Ramcharan, S., Faris, R., "Malignant Melanoma And Oral Contraceptive Use Among Women In California." p 247-52.

33   Beral, V., Evans S., Shaw, H., Milton, G., "Oral Contraceptive Use And Malignant Melanoma In Australia." *British Journal of Cancer,,* 1984; 50:681-85

34.   Love. op. cit. p. 134

35.   Paganini-Hill, A., and Henderson, V.W. "Estrogen deficiency and risk of Alzheimer's disease in women." American Journal of Epidemiology 1994;1140(3):256-2261

36.   Brown and Walker, op. cit. p. xiv

37.   Love. op. cit. p. 136

Chapter 18

1.   Lee, op. cit., p. 79

2.   The Burton Goldberg Group, *Alternative Medicine*, Future Medicine Publishing, Inc., Pulallup, Washington, 1993, p. 737

3.   Martin, op. cit. p. 118-119

Chapter 20

1.   *The Sunday Telegraph*, London, May 12, 1996

About the Author

Sherrill Sellman

Sherrill has, for the past 20 years, been conducting seminars, trainings and lectures both in the corporate and public sectors in the areas of women's health and personal empowerment, relationships, and mind/body healing. In addition she is a contributing writer to publications in Australia, New Zealand, Italy, Canada, United States, Germany and England.

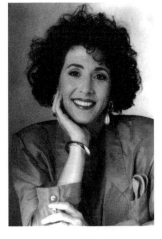

She is also a popular lecturer having been invited to speak at many conferences and special events. Sherrill resides in Melbourne, Australia where she also conducts a psychotherapy practice and rollerblades whenever possible!

For more information about Sherrill's programs, lectures and tours or to inquire further into the topics explored in her book contact:

Light Unlimited Productions

Locked Bag 8000 - MDC	Tel: (61 3) 9249-9591
Kew, Victoria 3101	Fax: (61 3) 9855-9991
Australia	email: golight@ozemail.com.au
	website: http://www.getwell.com

Index